CreateSpace Publishing, 2014

ISBN-13: 978-1505812145

Previously published by Lulu Press

Copyright ©2008 Diane Gross, All Rights Reserved: no part of this material may be copied by any process, including but not limited to fax, photocopy, computer scan or any other means for any purpose without the express written consent of the author or the author's designated representative.

Order book at www.createspace.com

Cover photograph by A. Lia Nester, CI and CT; Metro Referral Service

Sign Safely - Interpret Intelligently

A Guide to the Prevention and Management of Interpreting-Related Injury

Diane Gross, DOM (NM), L.Ac., Dipl. OM, CI and CT (retired)

"A practical and holistic approach to self-care for sign language interpreters. It encourages self awareness. The result is a win-win-win situation for the interpreter, consumer, and stakeholders. As more Deaf people gain access to all aspects of society, demands on interpreters will grow, so it makes perfect sense to incorporate an understanding of biomechanics in interpreting work. This is a necessary part of any interpreter training program and ongoing professional maintenance. The easy to follow tips are an excellent guide for well-being and optimal interpreting performance."

- Jacqueline Schertz
MS, CDI and Practicum Coordinator
ASL and Interpreting Education, NTID

Special Thanks

I am immensely grateful for the generous support of those who assisted me during various stages of writing this book. I would like to thank my wonderful husband, Richard, for his encouragement, his staunch love, and for his faith in me - as well as for the many, many hours he spent formatting this book. I am grateful to Dr. Alan Hurwitz for his support and kind endorsement. Thanks to Michael J. Rizzolo for his detailed editing, helpful suggestions, priceless business mentoring and friendship. I am deeply grateful to Marilyn Mitchell for her ongoing assistance as I wrote this book. She generously offered ideas, encouragement, and spent hours editing and re-editing. I appreciate Jacqueline Schertz for her support, gentle read and kind words. I could not have done it without them. I am indebted to interpreters across the country for all I have learned from them in almost two decades of conducting ergonomic workshops. A special thanks and tribute to my mentor, Dr. Michael Feuerstein, for everything he taught me about preventing and managing interpreting related injury. Thank you all.

Table of Contents

Introduction

Chapter 1- Interpreting Related Injury (IRI)

Chapter 2- Predisposing Factors to IRI

Chapter 3- Ergonomics of Interpreting

Chapter 4- Developing Low Risk Ergonomics

Chapter 5- Rest and Recovery Time

Chapter 6- Increase Your Interpreting Skills "Inventory"

Chapter 7- Exercise for the Interpreting Task

Chapter 8- Stress Management

Chapter 9- Pain Management

Chapter 10- A Plateful of Pain - or Energy?

Chapter 11- Self Care Using Acupressure and Self-Massage

Chapter 12- Work Stations

Chapter 13- Making Your Body Your Ally

Interpreter Bill of Rights

Note from the Author:
In writing this book I considered the question of whether I should write using the pronouns "you" and "your" or the more general pronouns of "we" and "our." My concern was that using the more direct terms of "you" and "your" might sound like I was lecturing, or even preaching. Yet the use of "we" and "our" often felt like the message of personal empowerment and individual responsibility for health and choices got lost. For example, the phrase "making *your* body your ally" has a very different feel to it than "making *our* bodies our allies." For me the first phrase is much more personal and powerful. As a result, I decided to use "you" and "your." My hope is that you, the reader, will find the information instrumental in helping you establish a long, enjoyable and healthy interpreting career.

Introduction

Interpreting-related pain is often seen as an unavoidable professional liability by sign language interpreters. Symptoms precipitated by the interpreting task are incredibly commonplace. In fact, a recent study conducted by Rochester Institute of Technology indicates that interpreters may actually be at greater risk of overuse injury than other professions commonly thought to be more susceptible.[1]

For years, during workshops on the prevention and management of interpreting-related injuries presented to interpreters, I have asked for a show of hands of those who believed that interpreters had to live with a certain amount of pain because of their work. It was not unusual for *everyone in the room to raise their hands!* This mindset is distressing to me.

If you believe pain and interpreting go "hand-in-hand," you are less likely to take action to mitigate the cause of your pain. I think *a much more useful approach is to recognize pain for what it is – a signal from your body that something needs attention.* Pain is an extremely important feedback mechanism, and it is important to pay careful attention to its message and to respond accordingly.

According to the Bureau of Labor Statistics, U.S. Department of Labor, injuries from repetitive motion continue to be the event with the highest median days away from work for all private industries (20 days). Musculoskeletal disorders accounted for 29 percent of all workplace injuries *requiring time away from work* in 2007.[2] This number doesn't include injuries *not* requiring time away from work, thus it appears this statistic may be just the tip of the iceberg. It is considered to be the leading reason for worker's compensation claims and lost wages in the United States today.

I originally became involved in working with sign language interpreters in the field of prevention and management of interpreting related injury in 1990 while working as a staff interpreter at the National Technical Institute of Technology (NTID). NTID's interpreting department was in crisis due to the number of work related injuries interpreters were experiencing. Out of 65 staff interpreters, 73% were receiving some form of work related accommodation due to symptoms. This was, of course, a major institutional crisis, in addition to the individual crisis for each interpreter involved.

In response to the emergency situation, NTID created a task force to determine remedial action. This task force involved a variety of stakeholders, including administrators, interpreters, interpreter educators and Deaf consumers.³ Collaboration between NTID and The Center of Occupational Rehabilitation (COR), University of Rochester Medical Center (URMC), created a comprehensive study of the problem.⁴

Factors potentially increasing the risk of injury to an interpreter were assessed. Scheduling concerns were analyzed and addressed, resulting in an overhaul of interpreter's work and recovery time ratio. This resulted in a better understanding of the ratio between the amount of work and recovery time. High work demand classes were staggered with classes demanding less physical and cognitive output.

Part of this study included dividing interpreters into two groups – those working with little or no pain and those working with pain. In the course of the study, each interpreter was required to interpret an already prepared Shakespearean class. The information was quite dense and at a fairly high level of complexity. Interpreters in each group were monitored utilizing sophisticated technology, in order to assess physiological response such as perspiration and heart rate, etc. Additionally, each interpreter was videotaped for later assessment by ergonomic experts to determine if there were any substantial differences in the ergonomics of those working with pain as compared to those working with little or no pain. It was found that there were significant differences.⁵

Following this study, NTID enlisted COR to provide training to interpreters on how to reduce the risk of Cumulative Trauma Disorder (CTD). CTD was the common terminology for overuse injury at that time. The training was presented over a period of ten weeks. While much of the more "generic" information was helpful, it was difficult for COR to make the pivotal ergonomic aspect relevant for interpreters. They:

- ♣ simply did not know sign language well enough to make their advice transferable to the task of interpreting;
- ♣ were unable to fairly assess which signs could be signed in a healthier ergonomic style, and which signs could not, and
- ♣ did not understand the nuances of non-manual markers and what was or was not a necessary part of the language and interpretation.

As a result, it soon became clear to NTID that a program needed to be developed *by an interpreter* that would be able to make the information relevant to interpreters.

Administration at NTID asked me to lead in the development of this project. I accepted the challenge and was privileged to serve as project coordinator and senior writer in the development of training for the prevention and management of CTD. This project required five years of working with experts in the fields of exercise physiology, occupational medicine, physical therapy, chiropractic, acupuncture, psychology, interpreting, and interpreter education.

During this time, I had the opportunity to be trained in the identification and remediation of general high-risk ergonomics. I have been able to successfully apply these principles to the interpreting field. For almost twenty years, I've been able to work with hundreds of interpreters from all over the U.S. Many have told me what they've learned in the workshop allowed them to continue their careers (visit my website at www.TerpHealth.com).

After leaving NTID, I continued conducting workshops for interpreters on prevention and management of sign language interpreting related injury with Ergotek, a company focused on providing ergonomic training nationally to interpreter. Eventually, I went back to school to become a Doctor of Oriental Medicine (DOM) in New Mexico, and a Licensed Acupuncturist (L.Ac.) in North Carolina. The materials that follow will utilize my expertise as a doctor of oriental medicine, as well my interpreting, training and ergonomic experience.

In this book the prevention and management of interpreting related injury will be explored from a multi-dimensional and often holistic perspective. Issues of ergonomics, scheduling, exercise, stress management, pain management, nutritional interventions, and self-care, including the use of acupressure and self-massage, will be addressed.

While this book can be helpful to those who are dealing with minor overuse symptoms, or for those seeking a sound preventative program, it is not meant to replace medical care for substantial, acute and/or chronic issues. It is also not meant to replace ergonomic diagnostic feedback by a qualified professional.

Chapter 1
Interpreting Related Injury (IRI)

Over the years various terms and acronyms have been utilized to describe the symptoms of injury due to "overuse." Some of the more common ones are Repetitive Motion Injury (RMI), Repetitive Strain Disorder (RSD), Overuse Syndrome, and Cumulative Trauma Disorder (CTD). When working with interpreters, I have chosen to call it Interpreting Related Injury (IRI), because it is clear that the repetitive aspect of interpreting is but one of the precipitators of symptoms. There are a number of things interpreters may face other than the ergonomics that can substantially impact the risk of injury. For example, interpreting a physical education class outside in 32 degree weather may increase the risk of injury much more than the "repetitive" motions involved during that assignment.

IRI refers to a variety of disorders typically associated with, but not limited to overuse, repetitive movements, poor ergonomics and/or insufficient rest or recovery time. There are other additional factors, such as anatomical or physiological predispositions, that may play a significant role in the development of an IRI that will be discussed.

IRI is related to the muscles, as well as nerves, tendons, ligaments, the neurovascular system and bones. Some of the more common IRI's experienced by interpreters are muscle soreness, tendonitis, tenosynovitis, carpal tunnel syndrome, De Quervains syndrome, and nerve impingement at various locations in the upper extremity. A short definition of each of these disorders is as follows:[6]

- **Muscle soreness:** Muscle soreness due to muscle exertion. This is often a result of lactic acid accumulation in the muscle or inflammation.

- **Tendonitis:** Inflammation of a tendon. This often happens as a result of repeated stress placed on the tendon due to overuse or poor ergonomics. The most common tendons affecting sign language interpreters are in the forearm.

- **Tenosynovitis:** Inflammation of the synovial membrane of a tendon. The most common area affected in interpreters is the wrist. Often this is related to excessive hand/wrist flexion.

- **Carpal Tunnel Syndrome (CTS):** Compression of the median nerve as it passes through the carpal tunnel in the wrist. There are many factors that can lead to CTS, including inflammation of the tendons in the carpal tunnel and a reduction in carpal tunnel space due to anatomical or physiological changes (e.g. bone spur, arthritis, overuse, hormonal imbalances, etc.).

- **De Quervain's Disease:** A type of tenosynovitis affecting the abductor muscles of the thumb and the side of the wrist.

- **Nerve Impingement:** Trapped, impinged or compressed nerves possibly due to anatomical or physiological changes.

Types of Pain Associated with IRI: Generally the first pain associated with IRI is an achy sensation. If it is not addressed it can worsen. The most common types of pain experienced by sign language interpreters are:

- Aching

- Redness and swelling of affected area

- Paresthesia, an abnormal prickling, tingling, burning, or crawling sensation on the skin.

- Numbness and loss of sensation

- Coldness

- Color changes (due to circulation problems)

- Reduction in range of motion (ROM)

- Joint impairment, including locking, clicking, triggering, popping, etc.

- Weakness, with accompanying reduction in ability to grip and hold things

How can you know if the symptoms you are experiencing are serious in nature, requiring medical intervention, or if they simply require a little extra rest and self-care? This is an important question.

You want to be sure to get medical attention if that is what's required. At the same time, with rising medical costs, if medical intervention is truly not necessary it can be helpful to know that as well! While there is no way that I can give "fool proof" or definitive advice, especially without the benefit of conducting a physical examination, there are some guidelines that can be helpful.

- **It is significant to determine if the pain is sudden or gradual can be significant.** A sudden onset of pain may point to an acute or traumatic cause. If you experience a sudden onset of pain, it is important to seek medical attention since this could indicate a soft tissue tear or injury of a more substantial nature. Gradual onset pain is often less serious, but still should be addressed in order to prevent worsening over time.

- **The quality of pain can help identify the source of the problem and determine if medical attention is warranted.** Dull, throbbing, or aching pain is often due to overuse or poor ergonomics. Generally this type of pain indicates muscles or soft tissue problems. In oriental medicine, different types of pain are important aspects of differential diagnosis

    o Muscle or soft tissue problems due to overuse can often be resolved simply by resting. Conversely, sharp pain, especially with movement, may be a sign of severe muscle spasms, or even a ligament, tendon, or muscle tear.

    o Burning, radiating and shooting pain, and/or tingling and numbness often indicate nerve involvement. Nerve involvement or tears require medical attention.

- **If the same movements always produce the same pain in the same place on the body it probably indicates that there is a specific injury that needs to be addressed, or that the activity may exacerbate the condition if continued.** This is an important consideration for interpreters because continuing to interpret in ways that precipitated symptoms, *while experiencing pain* will only produce more of the same.

- **Whether the pain is localized or referred may be telling.** When I was in school for oriental medicine my instructors would say "the injury is often *not* where it hurts." One instructor explained it with the adage, "It's not usually the bully on the playground that's the one complaining!" This is important because the goal is to remediate the *source* of the pain. Often you can know if the pain is referred or local, depending on if it is focal or diffuse. Focal pain tends to be caused by a problem in the local area. More diffuse pain tends to be referred from the actual area of injury. It can be helpful to look at a book or chart showing various "trigger points" on the body and the areas to which they refer pain.

- **If pain is coupled with other symptoms it may indicate a more complex or serious condition.** It can also be indicative of a connection between the two areas of the body. For example, Carpal Tunnel Syndrome (CTS) frequently has its genesis in the shoulder/neck region, or even the elbow.

- **What helps improve symptoms, and what causes them to worsen can be useful information?** There may be some joint or muscle dysfunction if movement makes it worse. If pain is worse with *passive* movement (i.e. someone else moves your arm for you and it hurts worse than when you move it yourself) that usually indicates ligament involvement. If pain shows no improvement with rest, medical attention should be sought. On the other hand, it is a positive sign if rest helps. If pain reappears quickly with resumed use, it could indicate the rest was insufficient, resumption of activity was too much - too fast, or it could mean the there is an underlying, unresolved injury that needs investigating.

- **If the pain responds positively to the application of heat or ice, it may indicate inflammation.** I often recommend anti-inflammatory foods and herbs such as turmeric, ginger, bromelain, and fish oil in this instance. I do not advocate the ongoing use of ice as a therapeutic modality for a chronic condition. I will address this later in the book.

- **How long the pain lasts is an important consideration.** We all have experienced short-lived pain such as sore muscles from time to time, but if the pain is relentless or chronic it needs to be addressed.

In a nutshell, if symptoms are sudden in onset, severe, sharp in quality, coupled with other significant symptoms, don't improve with rest, or are easily exacerbated and reproduced, an interpreter should receive a medical assessment. If pain has a gradual onset, is not intense, has an aching or throbbing quality, subsides with rest and improves with ice or heat, then the injury is probably fairly benign. Unless the injury is addressed it could become acute. Paying attention to your symptoms empowers you with information. It allows you the opportunity to make more informed choices about your health.

Chapter 2
Predisposing Factors to IRI

As depicted in Figure 1 below, there are a number of components that comprise the interpreting task.

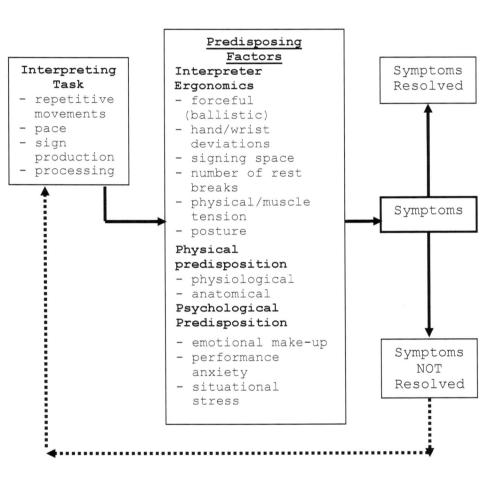

Figure 1: The Injury Cycle

©2008 Diane Gross, all rights reserved

While this is by no means a comprehensive list, it represents some of the essential elements of interpreting, which include:

- ♣ Repetitive Movements
- ♣ Pace
- ♣ Sign Production
- ♣ Processing

While the demands of the interpreting task may be impactful, the *significance* of the impact depends on the predisposing factors through which they are filtered. The greater the number of harmful filters, and the more severe the filters in question are – the greater the potential impact. The predisposing filters through which the interpreting task can pass include:

Interpreter Ergonomics: Chapter 3 will cover interpreting ergonomics extensively. It is an incredibly important aspect of staying healthy as an interpreter and a pivotal piece of the IRI-Interpreter connection, one that you can have control over.[7]

Physical Predisposition:

In order to approach interpreting in the safest way possible, it is important for interpreters to be aware of potential predisposing risk factors they may bring to their work. While not all of these risk factors may be alleviated, many can be addressed and resolved. Generally, predisposing factors fall into three categories. These include structural, physiological and psychological.

Anatomical Predisposition: The first predisposing factor that can increase the risk of injury is anatomical. Anatomical refers to the structural aspects of the body, including bone, vertebrae, tendons, and ligaments. Interpreting with a pre-existing anatomical condition may increase the risk of injury due to the stress interpreting places on the body. Anatomical issues may be the result of a congenital condition, an injury or a variety of other acquired disorders. While it may not be possible to reverse an anatomical predisposition, an interpreter may be able to make adjustments in his or her ergonomic approach to interpreting that can help minimize risk of injury. Type and length of assignments, as well as sensitivity to environmental and interpreting ergonomics, are important to consider when an anatomical predisposition is present. Examples of anatomical predispositions include:

Anatomical Predisposition:
This refers to specific anatomical or structural concerns that may increase the risk of IRI as a result of additional stress placed on the body. The interpreting task may tax the body in unique ways. These may include such things as:

- **Bone/spine abnormalities.** Examples include spinal subluxation, osteoporosis, bone spurs, etc.

- **Tendon/muscle/ligament abnormalities.** Examples include tendonitis, soft muscle injury, micro-tears, sprains, strains, spasms, etc.

- **Previous anatomical injuries or surgeries.** Examples include improperly healed broken bone, spinal fusion, pins or plates, etc.

Physiological Predisposition:
A physiological predisposition can refer to a wide variety of physical factors that can impact the risk of IRI. These may include:

- **Physical muscle tension**. Muscle tension can be caused by several things:
    - **Emotional tension.** Science has demonstrated that there is indeed a mind-body connection. If you are feeling emotionally stressed, then you *will* experience physical muscle tension. It is not possible to separate the two.

    - **Learned muscle patterns.** Muscles have "memory." These are habitual patterns of muscle movement, positioning, or levels of tension. The muscles of someone who constantly lives with significant levels of emotional and physical stress will "learn" or habituate tension. This is one reason a daily practice utilizing relaxation techniques can be so helpful.

Meditation and relaxation can help the body "unlearn" old, unhealthy patterns and assist in the development of new, healthier ones.

- **Static Loading.** Static loading occurs when muscles are held in an awkward or tense position for an extended period of time. This leads to muscle tension and spasm. Many people, for example, hold their shoulders up closer to the ears than necessary, as opposed to down in a relaxed position. This results in static loading the muscles in the arms, neck, or back, depending on which muscles are being stressed.

♣ **Hormonal imbalances.** Examples include:
- **Diabetes.** Diabetes is a disease in which the body is unable to produce or properly utilize insulin. Insulin is required for the conversion of food into the energy necessary for daily life. The function of the entire body and its ability to do work is compromised when insulin levels are not in balance.
- **Thyroid imbalances**. The thyroid regulates many functions in the body, including heart rate, digestion, physical growth, etc. If this hormone is out of balance, muscle weakness and damage can result.
- **PMS and pregnancy.** Many hormonal imbalances can occur around the menses and during pregnancy. One example that can impact the risk of IRI is that of fluid retention that often occurs at these times. This fluid can cause tissue to swell and put pressure on nerves, especially in the carpal tunnel.

♣ **Fatigue.** Fatigue can play a significant role in your physiological response to work. Rest and recovery time are important aspects of living a balanced life style. Your body, mind, and spirit needs time to recoup from your busy schedule and life.

♣ **Impaired or insufficient sleep.** It is absolutely essential that interpreters get enough quality sleep. Some experts believe that as much as 80% of your body's healing occurs during sleep. Deep, nourishing sleep is required if your body's cells are to fully recover from normal wear and tear, let alone heal from micro injuries that have resulted from the interpreting task.

- **Poor nutrition.** A balanced diet is necessary to provide the foundation with which to nourish, energize and repair the body. When these foundational nutrients are unavailable to the body, the chance for injury increases. Additionally, there are foods that can actually assist in the healing process, and others that can hinder the body's attempts to heal. These will be discussed later in greater detail.

- **Poor muscle strength, endurance and flexibility.** The level of your "fitness" impacts your risk of IRI. In interpreting each individual has to be mindful of their "work capacity." It is that level of work that can be safely managed without risk of injury. If you are always working at, or very near, your work capacity in a field requiring repetitive motions, then your chance of injury is increased. The easiest way to reduce your risk of injury is to increase your work capacity. The result is the ability to perform the physical demands of the interpreting task with greater ease. I do not plan to go into great detail in this book about more general strength, endurance and flexibility exercises since there are myriad sources on this topic available.

- **Poor general health.** This may be due to some of the factors already discussed, or some other cause such as disease. Regardless of what those factors may be, if there are overall health issues, then the risk of IRI may increase.

Psychological Predisposition:

Many years ago I thought high-risk ergonomics were the most impactful predictor of injury for a sign language interpreter. After more than 17 years of teaching workshops and performing diagnostics I have arrived at the conclusion that the psychological predisposition is the actually the most significant factor. It impacts the risk of injury at every level. It influences how you take care of yourself physically, how the interpreting task is approached, how you manage your pre-disposing factors, whether you advocate for yourself or accept unhealthy work terms and conditions, and how you respond if you experience discomfort from interpreting. Here are some examples:

- **External locus of control:** An external locus of control means to approach life as if it happens *to* you. An *internal* locus of control acknowledges that your personal choices determine how you experience life. An external locus of control can set an interpreter up for injury.

    For example, suppose you arrive at an assignment and find the chair has been positioned for your use during an all day job is a backless stool - with one leg missing. The stool is unstable and you are forced to carefully balance your weight every second in order to make sure that you don't tip over. Obviously I am being a bit facetious, but there have been times I have been presented with a situation that is not so different from this scenario! If you have an external locus of control you may accept the situation as inevitable and do your best to "work with it." In doing so, you set yourself up for injury.

    As a professional it is essential to have an internal locus of control. This will enable you to be resolute about what you need in order to do your work safely.

    A common situation interpreters often face is arriving for an assignment that requires two interpreters and finding, for whatever reason, they are by themselves for an all day job. An external locus of control would result in "sucking it up" and limping through the day regardless of resulting fatigue or pain levels. An internal locus of control would allow you to feel comfortable requiring some kind of accommodation that respects your physical safety needs and limitations. This could be contacting the organization through whom you are working and requesting support, working for only part of the scheduled event, asking for breaks every hour, or for another option that doesn't place you at risk of injury.

    If you are currently managing an existing injury, being externally focused can create a "why did this injury have to happen to me" mentality, rather than, "This happened, now what do I need to do in order to help myself in the best way possible?" An external locus of control keeps you stuck; while an internal locus of control helps you find and follow through with empowering choices

- **"Savior" mentality:** Sometimes interpreters find themselves constructing their lives and schedules around what they feel their consumer's need – to their own detriment. Sentiments such as, "If I don't interpret, then the Deaf person won't have anyone," and "I'm the only person they can understand," are not helpful.

    This kind of thinking and acting can easily cause you to live from a martyr stance, and may result in personal injury. This can sometimes feel like a difficult choice.

    Years ago I was personally dealing with an IRI while working in a college setting. The semester was only half over, but my pain levels were severe. I was struggling with feelings of guilt and the need to take care of myself because there truly were no other interpreters available! I remember my supervisor wisely saying to me, "While it would be very unfortunate, the worse case scenario is that the student may have to take the class again, but you only have two arms to last you for the rest of your life. Take care of them.

    You will not ultimately be doing your consumers a favor if you injure yourself to the point that you actually have to leave the interpreting field due to injury." I have never forgotten that feedback.

- **Stressful thinking:** When you engage in chronic stressful thinking it affects every bodily system. In addition to inhibiting blood circulation, upsetting your body's hormonal balance, and causing physical muscle tension, chronic stress can also affect the ability of your cells to receive nutrition from the food you eat! The cell receptors can actually get "hijacked" by the stress hormones. Obviously this impacts the ability of your body to repair and nourish itself.

    Additionally, when you engage in stressful thinking your cognitive abilities are compromised. This makes processing information while interpreting more difficult, which in turn can create more physical stress, etc. Furthermore, at a time when you must advocate for your own well-being, having full cognitive abilities would be important.

- **Perfectionism:** I think an "Achilles heel" of many sign language interpreters is demanding perfectionism in their work. This is not to imply that your goal should be anything less than producing work of the highest quality. However, perfectionism is an unfair and unrealistic demand. Have you, or someone you know, interpreted an entire assignment with great competence and accuracy…except for…one small (or large) mistake? We have all been there.

What is so fascinating is that interpreters often fixate on the one isolated mistake, rather than seeing it within the context of the amazing amount of skill and precision exemplified in the rest of the interpretation. While you should not be cavalier about making mistakes, or take your responsibility in the interpreting role lightly, it is okay to be human. Making mistakes does not make you a bad person – or bad interpreter. It simply means you are continuing to grow in your skills, knowledge and attributes.

I encourage interpreters to accept their current skill level, while working at increasing their skills with self-compassion and patience. I am concerned when those interpreters recently graduated from an interpreting program feel they should be as skilled as someone who has been in the field for 25 years. The level of tension and stress resulting from this expectation can increase the risk of getting an IRI.

Chapter 3
Ergonomics of Interpreting

There are essentially six high-risk ergonomic factors that sign language interpreters often employ. Research by NTID has shown that signing ergonomics are an important factor in one's risk of getting an IRI.

In many ways this is very good news. The ergonomics of interpreting are something over which each interpreter can have a significant amount of control. It may take focus, awareness and a plan to develop healthier ergonomic behaviors – but it can be done. I have seen hundreds of interpreters over the years do exactly that.

I do want to state here that each "high-risk" factor does in fact have an appropriate time and place. For example, if I am interpreting for two people who are screaming at each other, I will in all likelihood use the tool of force in my interpretation. If I am interpreting on stage, I will certainly have a large workspace. ***It is when high-risk ergonomic behaviors become the overriding style of interpreting that it is problematic.***

In order to begin to remediate any high-risk ergonomic factors it is vital to:

1) Be aware of what these risk factors are,

2) Determine whether or not you are engaging in any risk factors, and

3) Replace the high risk factor with a lower risk strategy.

All three of these steps are essential in order to reduce the risk of injury. While this may seem straightforward, it is not always quite so easy.

It seems to be very difficult to identify personal high risk interpreting ergonomics without help and without training. It's like trying to diagnose your own symptoms of disease using the Internet. My suggestion is to seek assistance from someone who can help you in pinpointing your ergonomic strengths and weaknesses.

The ergonomic factors to be discussed are:

- ♣ Appropriate use of force
- ♣ Healthy use of work-space
- ♣ Micro rest-breaks
- ♣ Hand/wrist positioning
- ♣ Physical muscle tension
- ♣ Posture

Force:

Appropriate use of force in interpreting is crucial. When I conduct ergonomic assessments, it is probably one of the risk factors I see most often. This style of interpreting is often called "ballistic" or forceful interpreting.

It is typified by:

- ♣ Signs with quick, abrupt starts (acceleration) and stops;
- ♣ Contact force which may, or may not, elicit sound;
- ♣ "Bouncing" quality to the signs;
- ♣ Extraneous movement of the whole body due to the force of signs.

In my estimation, the use of force to convey information is one of the most overused "tools" employed by sign language interpreters. It is often the primary methodology used to denote emphasis, intensity, volume, irritation, and anger. While it can be effective when used in conjunction with other strategies, if overused it can harm the body and skew the message. There are actually a number of non-manual markers that can be equally, or in some cases more effective than the use of force.

I remember a Deaf friend of mine being quite irritated with someone nagging him. He signed, "Finish!" to the person - not with force, but rather with almost *no* movement of the hand at all. The sign was produced very subtly and softly, *but the body language and facial expression spoke volumes!* The message was much more effective and clear than if he had employed the use of force. I think continually expanding your "interpreting inventory" allows you to better care for your body.

It's also interesting that an interpreter with a forceful signing style often appears angry while interpreting. This can substantially skew the message.

During workshops, I often show a videotape of an interpreter with a high force work style. Even though the speaker is clearly not angry, the interpreter appears quite angry. After the taping session, the interpreter we videotaped for the segment actually stated she *felt* angry while interpreting, though not angry going into the session. The movements had actually elicited an internal emotional response in the interpreter that matched the tone of her interpreting movements.

One of the challenges I present to interpreters who often use force is to consider the questions:

- ♣ "How little force is required to convey the necessary information with all its aspects and nuances?" Or,
- ♣ "If you weren't allowed to use any force at all to convey this information, how would you do it?"

This encourages the exploration and incorporation of other approaches as opposed to using force as a consistent default.

Workspace:

An interpreter's work-space, or work envelope can be too large or too small. There are unique challenges when either style is consistently utilized. If the work-space is too large, the muscles can become fatigued very quickly. The further away from the body the arms are held, especially for extended periods of time, the greater the risk of injury.

Consider this: If I hold a glass of water at arm's length, my muscles will tire much more quickly than if I hold the glass closer to my body. This is because the muscles are working much harder the further my arms are held from my body. It stands to reason that a consistently large work-space can significantly increase the risk of getting an IRI.

Likewise, an extremely small work-space, or one that is too high, can contribute to a variety of unhealthy ergonomic consequences. When signing is performed too close to the body, or in a very confined space, mobility of the upper arm is reduced. As a result, the wrists, and sometimes the elbows, become hyper-mobile in order to compensate.

Additionally, the shoulders tend to become hunched. When one's workspace is too high, it requires a tremendous amount of physical exertion to maintain the arm in the air. These elements can contribute to muscle spasms and straining of the wrist and elbow joints as they try to absorb the workload. This type of signing can result in micro-tears of soft tissue that over time can become cumulative.

A healthy workspace in which one should interpret is typically:

- **Height** = about waist level to the top of the head.

- **Width** = about shoulder width.

- **Depth** = extends to about three fourths of the fully extended arm.

Generally one should move fully within the workspace in a natural way as opposed to signing only within one quadrant or part of the space. As previously mentioned, there are situations in which a deviation from the "normal" work envelope is appropriate. An example of this is platform interpreting.

One caveat: it can be useful to avoid consistently interpreting in "high-risk" venues. If you do a lot of platform interpreting, it can be helpful to interpret at times in other environments requiring less space.

One setting I would like to specifically address is video relay service (VRS) interpreting. When conducting on-site ergonomic diagnostics at VRS call centers, I notice that Video Interpreters (VI's) typically sign with their chest as the lower border of their signing space. This is extremely high-risk interpreting.

When I mention this, I am generally told VI's must produce signs high enough to be seen on the screen. After working with numerous VRS call centers over the years I have not found this to be the case. With proper angling of cameras, monitors, chairs, etc, VI's *can* sign within a relatively normal workspace.

Micro rest breaks:

Micro rest breaks are different than rest and recovery time. Rest and recovery time refers to "down time" *between* interpreting assignments, affording your body time to recoup from the interpreting task. Micro rest breaks are those moments when you put one or both hands onto your lap if sitting, and to your side if standing - *while working*.

In the workshop demonstration tape we show an interpreting assignment in which 30 micro breaks were taken during a short three-minute interpretation! There are many opportunities for such "rests." For example, the non-dominant hand can almost *always* rest when the dominant hand is being used for finger spelling. Other opportunities for rest while interpreting include speaker pauses and effective utilization of visual aids.

Research conducted by COR and NTID shows that when the hand(s) is placed onto the lap, *even for microseconds* while interpreting, it significantly reduces post-interpreting symptoms of fatigue and pain. A question I am frequently asked by interpreters is, "But doesn't it take a lot more work to put the hands down for a micro-second, only to have to bring them *all the way back up* right away?" While that may *seem* to make sense, consider whether it is more fatiguing to hold a two pound weight out in front of you for 30 minutes straight, or to intersperse it with brief moments when your hand and arms are lowered.

One concern interpreters have regarding micro rests is whether it creates the impression the interpretation of the segment is finished. However, non-manual markers can be used as effective tools to convey information without the need to sign, thus allowing for additional opportunities to rest. These include utilizing body language and facial expression to denote that processing of information is still occurring.

I have observed many interpreters folding their hands and "resting" them on their chest or abdomen. These are not true rests. While they are certainly better than leaving the arms up and in the "ready" position, they are not as effective as lowering the hands into the lap for a full rest.

Hand/wrist positioning:

While some signs require a deviation of the hand and wrist area (such as HAVE), many can be produced without such deviations. The position of the hand and wrist should remain in neutral position as much as is possible.

According to the COR/NTID study hand/wrist deviations from neutral position were associated with greater pain and fatigue following an interpreting assignment. The number of hand/wrist deviations from neutral position in sign language interpreters places us squarely in the highest risk category for overuse injury.

There may be a number of underlying root causes for excessive hand/wrist deviations. Some that occur frequently are:

- ♣ Failure to rest the non-dominant hand during finger spelling. This leaves the hand hanging in the air and often leads to the hand sagging, causing a deviation from neutral position.

- ♣ Signing too close to the body. This creates a hypo-mobility of the upper arm and a hyper-mobility of the wrist.

- ♣ Signing in an excessively high work space. Signing too high will often directly lead to hand/wrist deviations. Simply lowering the sign eliminates the deviation.

- ♣ Development of an overly "relaxed" signing style. While being relaxed when signing is important, there does need to be a measured amount of control over the movement of the body.

- ♣ Lack of knowledge of how to sign particular signs without a hand/wrist deviation.

- ♣ Finger spelling in an awkward position. This is sometimes a result of not knowing the proper finger spelling position. However, some interpreters have been taught to finger spell with the palm position directly forward. This is a very high risk style for finger spelling. It creates a tremendous amount of tension from the wrist to the shoulder. Angling the palm position slightly to the non-dominant side eases the tension without losing clarity.

Finger 2: Spelling Position

Physical muscle tension:

If you are physically tense then you are more susceptible to an IRI. This is true for several reasons. First, since tense muscles are by definition less flexible, the risk for micro-tears increases, especially if there is concurrent forceful signing or excessive hand/wrist deviations. Increased muscle tension may also adversely affect the circulation of blood to the extremities.

Adequate blood supply to the arms is needed because of the work load. The blood carries the needed oxygen to the cells in the muscles and soft tissue that allows work to be done effectively and safely. Additionally, ample blood supply is essential to repair soft tissue that has been taxed during the interpreting task. It is vital that you approach interpreting with a relaxed and comfortable style. As mentioned in the previous chapter, some of the causes of physical muscle tension include:

- Emotional tension.
- Learned muscle patterns.
- Static Loading (holding muscles in a "static" position long enough to create physical muscle tension)

Posture:

It is important to feel comfortable and relaxed while interpreting. A proper posture can contribute to this end. Some of the reasons why a proper posture is vital to your work as an interpreter are:

- It ensures correct alignment of bones and joints, resulting in healthier muscles function.
- It reduces wear and tear on joints and ligaments.
- Static loading and strain and resulting pain and discomfort are reduced with proper posture.
- Fatigue due to the increased potential for inadequate circulation can be reduced.

Generally a "proper" posture can be described as follows:
- **Sitting:**
  - Feet flat on the floor.
  - Thighs parallel to the floor.

- Knees even with, or slightly higher than the hips.
- Back straight and shoulders comfortably back.
- Buttocks lightly touching the back of the chair.
- Normal curvature of the back.
- Both buttocks square on the chair, with weight distributed evenly.
- Legs ideally uncrossed; if legs are crossed, keep hips aligned on the chair and alternate the crossed legs.
- Change positions often to avoid static loading of muscles.

♣ **Standing:**
- Both feet flat on the floor
- Weight distributed evenly across foot
- Knees *flexible,* not locked
- Head held up
- Shoulder blades kept back
- Chin *slightly* tucked
- Knees directly over ankles
- Hips directly over knees
- Stomach slightly tucked into enhance natural curvature of the lower back
- Shoulders directly over hips
- Ears directly over shoulders
- The top of the head feel like it is being pulled upward.

Chapter 4

Developing Low Risk Ergonomics

General Strategies for Your Consideration

- **Set aside at least 10 minutes a day for practice**. When developing any skill it is important to practice. Developing low risk ergonomics is no exception. Just ten minutes a day can make a substantial difference in the quality and health of your ergonomics.

- **Find an interpreting model to observe, learn from and emulate.** It can be helpful to find someone who demonstrates low risk ergonomics in areas you are attempting to remediate. You can learn a great deal observing the various ways in which they produce signs and employ non-manual markers to convey information.

- **Use visualization techniques to imagine yourself signing in a low risk fashion.** This can be especially helpful to interpreters who are currently dealing with IRI and may be concerned with the additional stress to their extremities created by practice time. Visualization has proven to be extremely effective in the development and refinement of a wide variety of skills and can be employed to develop low risk interpreting ergonomics. The brain simply does not know the difference between what is real and what is imagined. This is why you can awaken from a bad dream with your heart pounding and dripping wet from sweat, or can feel a twinge of anxiety if you simply close your eyes and imagine a tarantula getting ready to crawl up your leg. Visualization can be utilized for the purpose of building healthier ergonomics and safer signing.

- **Eliminate high-risk signs one at a time.** Select one or two fairly common signs that you intend to sign in a low risk fashion *from this moment forward.* For example, you may decide to sign "people" without hand/wrist deviations from now on - no matter what. Once you have fully incorporated that change into your work style, you can target one or two more signs for remediation. In this way you begin to systematically shift your high risk ergonomic signing to that of a lower risk style.

- **Have a colleague observe your work and provide feedback.** This can be a helpful ongoing strategy. You receive feedback on your strategy as you work to make changes.

- **Increase your signing and non-manual "inventory."** This is so important. Interpreters often rely on the same "tools" with which to convey certain concepts, emotions or nuances. For example, forceful or ballistic signing is often utilized in order to convey intensity, anger or emphasis. In reality there are myriad ways in which you can convey these aspects via the use of effective non-manual markers. Exploring these can expand your skills and "interpreting inventory" significantly, thereby making you a much more versatile and effective interpreter.

- **During *practice time* strive for the "extreme opposite" of the behavior you are trying to remedy.** If you are seeking to develop a less forceful interpreting style, then strive for an extremely "soft" style during practice time. If you are focusing on learning to work with less tension, pretend your limbs are like wet noodles, etc. This doesn't mean you will be doing your interpreting *work* in this extreme fashion, but that you will garner the benefit of experiencing what "non-force" feels like, or what complete relaxation is like, and so on, when practicing.

- **Focus on changing your interpreting ergonomics during practice time, and slowly begin to incorporate these changes into your work.** Attempting substantial ergonomic changes during your actual interpreting work can result in a serious breakdown of your ability to process and interpret information accurately. It is much more effective to practice these new strategies prior to incorporating them into your interpreting work.

- **Give yourself time and permission to make mistakes and to move slowly.** Changing habituated ergonomic patterns is not a quick fix. It takes time and awareness. You *will* make mistakes. Beating yourself up for mistakes will slow your progress.

- **Relax and have fun.** Most of us entered this profession because we *love* the language and culture! At times we all need to get back in touch with the love and joy that initially drew us to this field.

Strategies for Healthy Signing Force

- **During practice time, sign to music.** Go with the flow and try to sign as "softly" as possible. This will support a rhythm and flow to your signing (as long as it is not acid rock!).

- **Visualize yourself signing underwater during practice time.** This helps to create a sensation of complete relaxation and buoyancy in your signing. It can help to reduce the force and speed with which you produce signs.

- **Learn additional ways in which to show grammar, emotion, tone and the mood of a message other then force.** Consistently interpreting with forceful ergonomics can actually skew the message significantly because it causes the interpreter to look angry and can misconstrue emphasis. Force is a powerful non-manual marker that can be powerful when utilized appropriately. If used just as a habitual style of interpreting it can misrepresent the intent and tone of the speaker.

- **Videotape your work and LISTEN to it.** Forceful signing is often, though not always, accompanied by sound. If you can hear your signs you can be sure you are signing too forcefully.

Strategies for Healthy Posture

- **Sit on a "no-slip" pad.** Sometimes interpreters begin their interpreting assignment with proper posture, only to start what I call the "slow slide." Within a few minutes their rear ends are hugging the edge of the chair and their backs are more horizontal to the seat of the chair than perpendicular. A no-slip pad, purchased in any department store, is a quick remedy.

- **Keep both feet on the floor.** This is ideal. However most interpreters prefer to cross their legs. If that is your style, I advice switching crossed legs frequently and keeping your hips square on the chair as opposed to leaning on one buttock.

- **Experiment with the "feel" of proper posture.** A healthy posture can take a while to get used to; however it can make a significant difference in your body's ability to sustain long periods of sitting or standing.

- **Practice optimum posture when not interpreting.** You cannot have poor posture in every other area of your life and expect to maintain a healthy stance while interpreting! It is important to foster good posture when you are not interpreting so that it becomes your natural default position.

- **Be aware of your head position.** Where your head goes, your body will follow. If your head is in alignment, your body will most likely follow suit.

Strategies for Healthy Hand/Wrist Positions

- **Incorporate more muscle groups into sign production.** I often see interpreters use as few muscles groups as possible when they interpret - in an effort to protect their arms. This can be counter-productive. In reality the more muscle groups that are employed, the less the risk of injury. This can be easily demonstrated by observing someone attempting to move a 200 pound stone. If he or she tries to do it alone it can be very difficult. However, with the help of two or three additional people the load becomes light. Ensuring the mobility and cooperation of all pertinent muscle groups while interpreting helps to minimize overtaxing one muscle group.

- **Experiment with the orientation and height of your hand, palm and fingers when producing signs.** This can affect whether a sign is produced with low or high risk ergonomics. For example, the sign "people" when signed near the head automatically results in a substantial hand/wrist deviation. When produced lower, below the chest the deviation naturally disappears.

- **Incorporate more rest breaks when your non-dominant hand is not in use.** The non-dominant hand inevitably will sag and result in a hand/wrist deviation if allowed to hang in mid-air while finger spelling with the dominant hand. Lowering the non-dominant hand onto the lap when finger spelling not only prevents deviations from neutral wrist positioning, but also provides momentary relief to the shoulder muscles.

- **Relax!** If your forearm muscles are tense this could cause a resulting hyper-mobility in the hand/wrist area. When one area of your body is less mobile, other parts of the body must become hyper-mobile to compensate. If the forearm muscles are tense, there is a reduction in movement of the forearm, resulting in hyper-mobility of the hand and wrist.

- **Sign in front of a mirror during practice time.** Observe your sign production carefully. It is challenging to notice or feel your own hand/wrist deviations. Observing your signs in a mirror or even on videotape can help you see deviations that you might not otherwise notice.

- **Place tape on the back of your hand and wrist area during practice.** This can increase awareness of times when you are signing with hand/wrist deviations.

- **Make sure your work-space is not too close to the body.** Sometimes interpreters sign close to the body in an attempt to protect sore upper arm or shoulders. However, this can create additional IRI symptoms over time. When the work-space is too close to the body, the upper arms and forearms become less mobile resulting in hyper-mobility of the hand/wrist area.

Strategies for Reducing Tension

- **Take deep breaths often.** In the chapter addressing stress management I detail the many benefits of breathing. One of the payoffs is a significant reduction in both mental and physical tension. There are many missed opportunities to breathe while interpreting.

- **Use the speaker's pauses as a cue to LOWER your shoulders.** When combined with breathing, lowering the shoulders can make a huge difference in the levels of post interpreting pain and fatigue. Many people can easily and quickly lower their shoulders with a moment of awareness. What is interesting is that if you can lower you shoulders, then you are tense Otherwise your shoulders would not have been elevated. Many people carry much more tension than they are aware of. Using this simple exercise can help bring awareness and help you to release some of that tension.

- **While maintaining proper posture, purposefully get in a very relaxed physical position when interpreting.** If your body is relaxed, your mind will follow. The mind-body connection is powerful. It is not possible to be physically tense, while at the same time mentally relaxed. Likewise you can't be mentally tense and physically relaxed. If you find yourself feeling tension, then a simple remedy is to relax and release your muscles. There is a quick method called "progressive relaxation" that is very effective. Simply begin by relaxing your feet muscles and work up your body. As you notice a tense muscle or muscle group simply mentally release them. As you do so, not only will your physical tension lessen but so too will your mental stress.

- **Practice relaxing at least 10 minutes daily.** The benefits of doing so are well documented. Sometimes life is busy and filled with noisy distraction. It is easy to habituate a state of stress and tension. Relaxing for even a few minutes a day can help bring you back to a state of awareness and calmness. I personally meditate for one hour each morning before starting my day. I am then able to make decisions and perform my daily tasks from a calm center.

- **Prepare for the assignment and use professional discretion when accepting assignments**. Interpreters sometimes indirectly contribute to their own experience of stress by not utilizing professional discretion when accepting assignments. There is a big difference between honing your skills by taking on an assignment that is difficult, and accepting one that is completely beyond your abilities. Deliberately stepping into any situation for which you do not have the resources can lead to frustration and tension.

- **Limit caffeine prior to assignment.** Caffeine is a stimulant and can create substantial tension when used in excess. Prior to an assignment may not be the best time to consume substances that increase tension.

- **Eat foods that nourish your nervous system.** The importance of a healthy diet cannot be overstated. It absolutely affects your risk of IRI in a variety of ways, only one of which is to provide the nervous system with what it needs in order to maintain a sense of composure and calmness.

Strategies for a Healthy Work Space

♣ **Sign in front of a mirror on which you have drawn an "interpreting space box" for yourself.** This will enable you to observe how effectively you work within a healthy signing space. Do you have many excursions outside of the space drawn on the mirror, or do you under-use the space?

♣ **Videotape your practice times and observe your progress with a proper interpreting space drawn on the screen.** Again, this will allow you to clearly see how effectively you are utilizing a normal work space.

♣ **Experiment with ways to sign in a healthy interpreting work space with the *careful* use of barriers such as doorways or walls.** If you under utilize the space, then attempt to *slowly and carefully* expand the use of your sign space. If you are signing in too large of a space, then create an obstruction that limits your ability to sign too large. This strategy should be used with caution and very slowly in order to ensure you don't accidentally hit yourself or jam a finger or thumb on a doorway or wall.

♣ **Be aware of the proper position for finger spelling.** This is extremely important! A large number of interpreters finger spell with their arm and hand positioned improperly. This causes excessive stress of a substantial nature on the entire upper extremity. The proper position for finger spelling can be found quite easily. Place your finger spelling hand in a relaxed position in your lap and then, without moving your elbow, just lift your hand. The orientation of the palm will actually be slightly diagonal. There is no need to force your palm outward to face the Deaf person to whom you are interpreting. Most Deaf people never fingerspell in this fashion. If, for some reason, you must ensure the palm is faced outward, then just slightly shift your body so that the palm is clearly visible.

♣ **Practice small body-shifts.** Large body shifts are generally not necessary unless interpreting on stage. Body shifts that are too large can cause you to go outside of a healthy interpreting work space and compromise your posture.

Strategies for Incorporating Rest Time During an Assignment

- **Use finger spelling as a cue to rest your non-dominant hand.** As mentioned above, the non-dominant hand should always be placed down and into your lap if sitting and by your side if standing when finger spelling. Research indicates that increased numbers of one and two handed micro rest breaks while interpreting are associated with less pain and fatigue afterward.

- **Have someone count your one-handed and two-handed rest breaks during your practice time.** It is amazing to see how these small micro-second rests can be utilized.

    People ask me, "Isn't it more work to put the hand down and then have to bring it all the way back up again?" At first blush that may seem logical. However, consider the muscle fatigue you would most likely experience if you held your arm straight in front of you without rest for an hour compared to that you might experience if you periodically put your hand down – even if just for a moment.

    When one or both hands are lowered, there is a corresponding relief to all of the adjacent muscle groups. Additionally, putting your hands down - even for a second or two - minimizes "static loading" of the muscles. Static loading occurs when muscles are not allowed relief, and the results are tension and spasms.

    An example I often use is that of holding a water bottle out at arm length. If held there for ten minutes, the arm will tire significantly. If the arm is permitted to fall for even a second or two, the experience will not be close to the same level of fatigue. The dynamics are the same with interpreting.

- **Have a colleague or team partner "cue" you to rest during your assignment.** I have seen interpreters work for as much as an hour or more without putting their hands down once. When this pattern of interpreting has been habituated it can take time and focus to initiate change. Feedback and cuing from someone can be helpful.
- **Use speaker pauses effectively:** Take advantage of speaker pauses to rest. Obviously if you are allowing yourself time to "process" information there will be a lag time between the speaker pause and your rest. However the opportunity is still there.

Chapter 5

Rest and Recovery Time

In addition to incorporating micro-rest breaks, appropriate rest and recovery time is an important aspect for the prevention of IRI. If the body is not being given sufficient recovery time, the risk of injury increases. Your body needs time to rest. IRI generally occurs as a result of multiple micro injuries incurred while interpreting. Your body needs time to repair and heal itself. Pacing yourself and your schedule, and building in adequate time to heal should be a primary professional consideration. Each person has different needs, but some good guidelines are:

- **Ensure that you are interspersing heavier and lighter assignments**. This guarantees greater balance in your work life and schedule. Certainly there may be times when a special "high demand" assignment lasts a number of days. However such assignments should be extraordinary. Exceptions do happen, but you must take care to ensure that the exceptions do not become common practice as you frame your schedule. Each assignment should be considered within the larger scope of the "heavier followed by lighter" principle.

- **Work with team interpreters for long assignments (over two hours unless the assignment is light**. I know this can be a challenge; however working for long periods of time alone can greatly increase the risk of IRI. This is an area I believe you need to professionally insist on as a part of ensuring a safe work environment

- **Advocate for your scheduling needs.** This too can be "sticky." One of the most common things interpreters say to me is that their employers will not accommodate their needs. I have spoken with interpreters who have had three carpal tunnel surgeries because the organization for which they worked would not "allow" them to have team interpreters, or insisted that they interpret from 9:00 AM – 3:00 PM without reasonable breaks. While I do not advocate approaching things with an adversarial attitude, I also do not advocate laying your body on the altar of interpreting to avoid conflict.

I encourage interpreters to place their needs first and foremost with scheduling. You are not doing anyone a favor if you create a disability. Then you will not be able to interpret *at all!* Interpreters are not to be martyrs. It is vital to use discretion when accepting assignments because taking care of your body by maintaining needed appropriate rest and recovery time is part of professionalism.

♣ **Don't leave pain unaddressed.** If you are hurting, sore or feeling achy, your body is sending you a signal that you need rest and recovery time. Continuing to engage in the activity that caused the initial symptoms, will only exacerbate the symptoms! It's like running with a sprained ankle. Everyone knows that running with a sprained ankle is a bad idea. It needs rest in order to heal. If you continue running while it is injured, the ankle will likely get worse. The same is true with issues regarding your upper extremities. Allowing your body to recuperate is one of the most powerful things you can do to reduce the risk of, and/or manage an existing IRI.

Chapter 6

Increase Your Interpreting Skills "Inventory"

Increasing your interpreting inventory expands your technical skills as a sign language interpreter, and it also may help provide you more ergonomically safe alternatives. In essence, it gives you the power of choice. Some helpful ways to increase your interpreting skills inventory include:

- **Find one or more "models" of ASL from which to learn.** This can be especially helpful if you are able to find someone who exhibits a low risk style of interpreting in the area in which you are focusing. For example, if you sign too forcefully, find someone who is highly skilled technically, and yet exhibits a softer ergonomic style. Watch how they move. Observe the non-manual markers they employ in order to relay information that you might have unnecessarily used force to convey. Notice the signs they produce with a neutral hand/wrist position as compared to ones you may sign with excessive wrist movement. Spot opportunities for micro rest breaks that were capitalized on, along with how speaker pauses were managed. See how they utilize visual cues in the environment.

- While the intent is not to become an interpreting "clone," there is much we can learn from one another. Gleaning from one another's strengths gives us the opportunity to learn and grow by capitalizing and building on the experience and knowledge of others.

- **Include a minimum of five-ten minutes a day (or 30 minutes a week) to focus on skill development, including healthy ergonomics, as part of your professional development plan this year.** (Side note: I hope each of you do have a yearly professional development plan for yourself! It can make all the difference in the world regarding whether you excel or are mediocre in your field. It can also greatly impact your risk of IRI.). Just a few short minutes every week can add up quickly. Just ten minutes every day, five days a week, adds up to over 43 hours over the course of a year. You can learn a *lot* in 43 hours!

♣ **Commit to learn *and use* at least one new way of signing something every day.** Look for opportunities to incorporate what you learn into your work during the course of the day so that it becomes a part of your interpreting inventory. This can be a great way to add a little creativity into your work. It can be fun to see how many times you can utilize a new skill or sign. Of course it must be appropriate to the setting and interpretation or it should not be utilized. The goal is for the newly learned signs and skills to augment your interpretation, not to skew it just because you want to "try out" your new sign or skill.

Chapter 7

Exercise for the Interpreting Task

This chapter includes a variety of aspects, including warming up and cooling down prior to and following interpreting, as well as increasing physical strength and endurance.

As previously mentioned, I do not intend to delineate specific strength and endurance exercises because there are a number of wonderful programs already available to the general population that can be utilized by interpreters. I do, however, strongly recommend that *every* interpreter make keeping fit a high priority.

It is essential to develop the necessary strength and endurance for the interpreting task. The risk of injury significantly increases when muscles are not strong enough to handle the task of interpreting. Interpreting requires a great deal of stamina, and one of the easiest ways to decrease the injury risk is to increase physical strength.

Stretching

One aspect of exercise to address here is that of stretching. I am not a proponent of the most common approach to stretching in America today. It generally involves stretching the muscle to the utmost (or very nearly) for anywhere from a few seconds to a few minutes. I have treated many patients who have tried to increase their range of motion and flexibility utilizing this approach. I encourage them to try is a softer approach to stretching.

Often muscles that could benefit from some lengthening are tight and tense, which is why they need to be stretched. The problem is that people stretch muscles like rubber bands. When you stretch a rubber band it gets tight! So I believe that to stretch a "tight" muscle in a "tight" way leads to a muscle memory of tightness.

Sometimes people may even find there is a shortening of the muscle fibers in response to stretching techniques that are too aggressive. This is the body's efforts to protect a muscle it perceives as being over stretched. The muscles "feel" attacked when stretched in this way.

I have seen *dramatic* positive results with a much softer approach. For example, I had a patient who was training for a marathon. This individual had run many marathons in the past, but this time found himself running with an 8 out of 10 pain level during training (0 is no pain, 10 is the worse pain possible). He had been trying to stretch his hamstrings in the typical fashion; however, things were simply getting worse after 4 months. He had been receiving acupuncture from another practitioner and decided to come to see me at the recommendation of a friend.

In addition to acupuncture treatments, I suggested he try a different approach to stretching that I call "moving into softness." The stretching movements are the same, but performed with a different intensity and focus. Instead of trying to move the muscles into the biggest stretch possible, I suggested that if it "felt" like a stretch he was *going too far!* I explained that if he made sure he did not stretch" beyond the point that he could *completely* relax his hamstring muscle, then his muscle would actually begin to "let go" and lengthen. I told him that he could move a little further into the stretch once his muscles got used to that position, as long as he was still able to keep his hamstring perfectly relaxed in the new position as well. Within 1 week he was running with 50% less pain, and within three weeks he was running without pain.

Often people are able to stretch just as far as when they were "cranking" the stretch without the rebound, if they are willing to just take a little more time to do so.

Warming up and cooling down prior to and following interpreting is a significant part of professional self-care. When I was at NTID the Center for Occupational Rehabilitation (COR) compared the demands placed on a sign language interpreter's body to the demands placed on a dancer's body. Just as a dancer would *not even think* of dancing without warming up and cooling down, so too should interpreters give equal importance to doing so.

The same exercises can be done for both warming up and cooling down. Let's look at the function of warming up and cooling down separately:

Warming up

Gentle warming-up of the entire body is optimal. Warming up helps prepare the muscles, tendons, ligaments and blood vessels for the interpreting task. It increases flexibility and circulation to the entire body, including the upper extremities. This greatly reduces the risk of injury.

Caution with Warming-up: Warm up movements should be measured and performed with *control.* This is extremely important, *especially if you are experiencing current IRI symptoms!* Uncontrolled movements and abrupt gesticulations such as shaking the hands, or ballistic, forceful movements do not allow the body time to adjust and can strain soft tissue and joints.

Systemic Warm up: A systemic warm up can be as simple as a brisk walk from the parking lot or isometric exercises. The goal is the get your blood circulating, resulting in more efficient oxygenation of the whole body, including the arms and hands. If you try to warm up the hands and arms in isolation, without a total warm up, the effect is short lived and incomplete. Your body works as a whole unit. Sometimes I see interpreters trying to warm up by running their hands under hot water. While this can certainly be helpful if you are coming in out of freezing temperatures, do not be fooled into thinking that it has made your muscles ready for work. It can help create a short term, localized effect, but if the circulation of the whole body is not stimulated, the circulation of blood to the hands and arms *will* be short lived.

Targeted Warm-up: After a systemic warm up, targeted, smaller and exaggerated movements may be performed that mimic signs to specifically warm up the muscles used in interpreting. This includes gentle stretches, leisurely signs and finger spelling. The goal is to increase the mobility and flexibility of the hands and arms for interpreting.

Cooling Down

Cooling-down, though often ignored, is as important as the warm-up. It allows the body to remove residue waste products produced during the work of interpreting, such as lactic acid. These waste products are by and large responsible for the soreness that results from exercise performed without the benefit of cooling down. Cooling down also allows the body to gently return to homeostasis. It helps to expedite the recovery process since residual waste products impede healing.

Chapter 8
Stress Management

Many people in the health care field now believe that stress plays a greater part in the risk of injury and disease than previously thought and can significantly impact the body's ability to heal. It affects brain function, cardiovascular system, nervous system, endocrine system, and digestive system, including the ability to assimilate nutrients from the foods eaten. All of this, of course, impacts the risk of IRI.

Feeling emotionally stressed is an experience we all share at one time or another. From an Oriental Medical perspective emotional stress can certainly create imbalance in the body, which makes it susceptible to injury, illness and disease. The Neijing, the oldest and most authoritative Oriental Medical text, says that overindulgence in emotions can create imbalances in the body.[8]

Unbalanced emotions can lead to impairment of Qi (pronounced "Chee"), Blood and Yin. Qi is essentially the body's energy system. If Qi does not flow freely, or is depleted or impaired in some way, emotions will be negatively affected. Blood is considered to be the physical basis for the "Shen," or Spirit, which includes the emotional and mental aspect of your life. If there is disharmony with the Blood, there isn't the needed foundation for healthy, balanced emotions. Yin is essential to moisten and nourish your body and to "anchor" your more "Yang" or aggressive energies.

Just as the harmony of Qi, Blood and Yin is necessary for emotional well-being, your physical health may be affected, either negatively or positively, by your emotions. Repressed, or over indulged emotions and stress, such as anger, mania, sadness or worry, can result in illness. In the same way, illness and disease may disrupt emotional balance. In order to reduce stress it can be helpful to maintain daily practices designed to reduce stressful thinking and increase a positive mindset.

From a western perspective the experience of stress also has been demonstrated to impact your risk of IRI. It increases muscle tension, decreases blood flow to the extremities, increases the body's autonomic functions, decreases mental function and increases pain levels.

There are many effective methods for reducing the experience of stress in your life. It is not my intention to address each method in depth. I have addressed some of them with varying levels of depth below:

- **Acupuncture:** Acupuncture is an incredible modality for balancing the energies of the body, resulting in a reduction of stressful feelings. It has been shown to stimulate endorphins and other chemicals in the body that elevate mood, assist in healing and promote sound sleep.

- **Meditation.** There are many forms of meditation that can be helpful. Find the specific "style" that best suits your needs. The goal is to schedule time daily when you are able to quiet your mind and enter a state of calmness. Some people experience this as connecting with their "Higher Power," while other people simply see it as an opportunity to momentarily leave the busyness of life and sit quietly. Whatever it means for you is perfectly fine, but experts in the health field overwhelmingly agree that daily meditation can be an extremely helpful addition for those seeking to reduce stress.

- **Eat to feel good.** Your brain literally uses the food you eat as the raw material from which to make the chemicals it needs to help you feel good. Chapter 9 is dedicated to the topic of nutritional interventions to manage pain and to support emotional health.

- **Practicing a positive mindset.** It has been said that situations cannot cause stress, but feelings of stress are the result of stressful thinking. Many psychotherapists believe emotions are actually a result of thought. This means that thoughts give birth to emotions rather than the other way around. If you are feeling sad, the sadness was generated by a specific thought.

    The same would be true of all emotions, including feelings of anger, frustration, joy, excitement, etc. The idea is that if a situation can be stressful in and of itself, then everyone would experience stress if exposed to the very same situation. This is not usually the case. For example, one person interpreting for the President of the United States might feel extremely stressed, while someone might be energized and exhilarated by the challenge.

    If thoughts truly do generate emotions, then it may be prudent to be aware of what your thoughts are and to practice and nurture those that encourage positive and empowered emotions.

- **Lower your tolerance for stress.** At first blush this may seem a bit counter intuitive; however, it can help to greatly reduce your experience of stress. It is a matter of honoring the need for a balanced life, as well as having a keen sense of the stressors in your life. Often people try to power through situations, or just "suck it up" rather than focusing on initially setting healthy boundaries. If you feel too busy and overwhelmed in your daily life, you may be tolerating too much stress.

It is important to recognize and address potential stressors. Of course we all need to develop internal fortitude and strength in the face of adversity. However that is very different than allowing the fodder for stress to muddy your life. Consider, for example, how much frustration you might experience while interpreting if you accepted an assignment for which you truly did not have the skills to perform. You most probably would experience feelings of stress - the same stress prevented by simply turning down the assignment. It is making a conscious choice to not accommodate avoidable stressors in your life.

Lowering your tolerance for stress is a pro-active approach to experiencing more peace and balance in your life. Placing a high premium on living a balanced lifestyle will prompt you to take appropriate action when something threatens to compromise that balance.

- **Get adequate sleep.** Sleep is a vital ingredient for maintaining health and to enhance healing. A substantial amount of healing actually takes place during deep sleep. Symptoms mimicking fibromyalgia and chronic fatigue syndrome can be elicited by denying even a few nights worth of deep sleep. One reason for this is that human growth hormone peaks during deep sleep. Because sleep difficulties have become such a scourge in American society, I often advise people to maintain what is commonly known as "health hygiene."

Good sleep hygiene contributes greatly to consistent and restful, healing sleep. Some aspects of sleep hygiene include:

  o Try to go to bed and get up at the same times every day. This allows your internal clock to "set." Your body will start to get tired as you approach bedtime when you develop a pattern.

  o Try to schedule sleep times aligned with the natural rhythms of nature. This means being awake during the daylight hours and sleeping at night.

- Lighten up your morning with some sunshine. Light helps reduce levels of melatonin in the brain (the sleep hormone) and increases serotonin. This too will help to regulate your hormones for optimal sleep.

- Be careful of too much caffeine intake, especially in the afternoon and evening.

- Avoid alcohol within four or five hours prior to bedtime. While alcohol may help some people fall asleep faster, it tends to cause a delayed sleep disturbance.

- Avoid eating heavily in the evenings. It has been said that if you eat late at night you will either digest well or sleep well- but not both. Heavy, greasy and spicy foods are of particular concern.

- Do not do anything in bed other than sleep or sex since you want your brain to associate bed with sleep, not television.

- Engage in calming activities prior to bed. Relaxation techniques such as deep breathing can help the body decompress from the day. Television and computer work can actually stimulate the brain.

- Avoid vigorous exercise within two hours of going to bed.

- If you have trouble "turning off your mind," try soaking just your feet in very warm water for 15 minutes prior to bed. In Chinese medicine this is believed to bring the energy down and out of the head. I have seen this make a real difference for people.

- Make sure your sleeping environment is comfortable, quiet, dark and at a moderate temperature.

- Establish a ritual prior to bedtime. This sends your brain a signal to also prepare for sleep.

- If you do not fall asleep within a half hour, get out of bed and read a book (not a white knuckle thriller…) until you feel sleepy, then go back to bed.

- Do not try to go to sleep. Allow yourself to "daydream." Going to sleep is a natural process. Trying to fall asleep actually will cause tension that prevents the natural process.

♣ **Breathe:** Breathing is vital to life! It supplies your body with oxygen, and it also helps eliminate toxins and metabolic waste products, including accumulated carbon dioxide. Literally *every cell* in the body needs sufficient oxygen to function healthily. This is important because *decreased* levels of oxygen contribute greatly to fatigue and inhibit the natural ability of the body to heal from injury and disease. Some benefits of deep breathing that directly reduce the risk of IRI for sign language interpreters risk include:

- It is essential for healthy brain function. This greatly affects your ability to process information in a clear and helpful way while interpreting.

- It enhances your body's ability to recover and heal from injury and disease.

- It helps your body eliminate toxins.

- It assists in the digestion of food and assimilation of nutrients from the foods you eat.

- It oxygenates the nervous system, which interfaces with every system of your body.

- It provides oxygen to the glandular and hormonal systems. This is important because some hormonal problems can increase the risk of IRI.

- It affects the parasympathetic nervous system, resulting in more physical muscle relaxation. This can directly reduce the risk of IRI.

- It reduces anxiety, which for sign language interpreters is a risk factor for IRI.

- **Movement Therapies:** There are many movement therapies that can assist in the reduction of stressful feelings. Three of my favorite include:
  - **Yoga:** Yoga, as a method, is famous for reducing stress, as well as stretching and relaxing the body. I believe it can be a helpful modality if approached with care and wisdom. I have been practicing yoga for more than 25 years and have noticed that sometimes people can get overly ambitious and hurt themselves with stretches and stances for which they are ill prepared. If you choose to do yoga, I encourage you to find an experienced, licensed yoga instructor for instruction.

  - **Feldenkrais Method:** Feldenkrais is great for sign language interpreters! It helps you learn to move with more ease and freedom, to carry less physical stress, and to recognize and stop moving in ways that cause pain. It utilizes gentle movement and focused awareness of the body and its movement as a medium to improve physical function, enhance fluidity and ease of movement, along with an increased range of motion. I have also seen it dramatically reduce pain and tension resulting from imbalanced and overly stressed muscles.

    The Feldenkrais Method utilizes principles of physics and proper ergonomic biomechanics in its carefully prescribed movements. These movements are intended to bring your attention to the areas of your body that are unbalanced due to lack of awareness. As you move through the sequence of movements, you learn new ways of moving and actually begin to exchange old neuromuscular patterns for new healthier ones. I typically recommend Moshe Feldenkrais' book entitled Awareness through Movement for people interested in learning more about The Feldenkrais Method.

  - **Tai Chi:** Often called Tai Chi Chuan, this is an ancient form of self defense originating in China at least 2000 years ago. It is sometimes called "meditation in motion" due to the fact that it helps to connect the mind and body through its gentle, dance-like movements that are coordinated with the breath. I have noticed that this particular form of movement "therapy" is especially helpful for sign language interpreters because it helps interpreters learn to move their body through space softly, in alignment and with all parts of the body working together in harmony. Tai Chi, when practiced regularly helps to significantly reduce stress, while increasing flexibility, energy, strength and coordination.

- **Qi Gong:** Qi Gong is a method designed to help balance and strengthen the Qi, or energy of the body, thereby assisting in the natural healing process. It is extremely powerful and effective.

Chapter 9
Pain Management

Pain management includes a wide scope of strategies that should be considered when dealing with an existing IRI. Certainly everything mentioned in this book has a place as part of a comprehensive pain management program. However, some modifications may be needed in order to accommodate an injury. For example, though the preventative strategies listed may be useful when employed in a pain management program, there is a caveat.

It is *absolutely vital* to determine if the extent or severity of your injury precludes interpreting safely at all. You may need a break in order for your body to heal. If you *can* realistically continue to interpret with accommodations, it may be necessary to outline what those accommodations need to be. Some general things to consider when dealing with existing pain or injury include (note: some of these have already been discussed as part of a comprehensive prevention program, but deserve special mention here as well):

- **Seek assistance from your health care practitioner regarding the status of your condition.** It is important to determine whether you can safely continue to work or if you need recovery time. Continually stressing an injured extremity can potentially lead to permanent consequences. It is no different than continuing to run on a sprained ankle. There is an appropriate time for everything, including time for healing and recovery.

- **Include prevention and management of IRI in your annual professional development goals.** Prevention and management is equally as important as developing technical and language skills as an interpreter. It helps you to focus attention on interpreting safely.

- **Deal with IRI symptoms immediately.** Too often people ignore initial symptoms in hopes that they will miraculously go away. In reality, if symptoms are not dealt with they will generally become worse. If, while injured, you approach interpreting in the same manner that precipitated injury with a sustained injury, it will exacerbate the problem.

- **Balance extracurricular activities with your work.** Watch for hobbies that are of a repetitive nature. This does not mean that you cannot continue to do the things you love; it simply means you need to balance the various aspects of your life so that you can maintain your health.

- **Watch for high-risk ergonomic behavior in your everyday activities as well as in your interpreting.** You can be sure that any high-risk interpreting ergonomics show up in other areas of your life. If you sign forcefully, for example, then you probably do many things in your life in a forceful and ballistic manner. This would include such activities as typing, writing, chopping food, etc.

- **Use stress reduction and pain management strategies.** Your experience of pain is strongly influenced by our levels of stress and perceptions of what the pain means for you. Stressful feelings affect your body in significant ways, including affecting your circulatory and endocrine, or hormonal systems. Additionally, the meaning you assign to your pain impacts the experience of pain. For example, my experience of pain will be different depending on whether I believe my stomach pain is due to cancer as opposed to the fact that I ate too much.

    Remember, stress also has some bearing on your ability to absorb nutrients. Chronic stress can result in stress hormones "hijacking" nutrient receptors on the cells. This can of course impact the body's ability to repair and heal.

- **Soak in Epsom Salt.** Soaking in magnesium sulfate crystals, commonly known as Epsom Salt, can assist with pain management. Magnesium sulfate is absorbed easily through pores of the skin and can benefit your body in a variety of ways. First, Magnesium is essential for the maintenance of appropriate calcium levels in the blood.

    Calcium is necessary for the conduction of electrical impulses in the body, directly impacting the function of every cell and bodily system. Magnesium is also well known as the "relaxation mineral." It is a natural stress reliever - both physically and emotionally. Additionally, Epsom Salt has the capacity to remove toxins from your body, including heavy metals via reverse osmosis. The result can be a reduction in muscle pain and inflammation.

Epsom Salt also delivers sulfates (*not* sulfites) to your cells. Sulfates are more easily absorbed your skin than through the food you eat. Sulfates assist in forming brain tissue, joint proteins and the lining of the digestive tract. Sulfates have also been shown to help detoxify the body.

The one important caution when using Epsom salts is that it can dry out the skin if overused. I generally recommend ½ cup in the bath, 1-2 times a week to start. This will enable you to gauge how your skin is going to react. This can be increased as needed and tolerated. If your skin starts to dry out, then reduce the amount, or take a break from using it for a while.

- **Use Ice sparingly and with caution.** A question I am often asked by patients with chronic pain resulting from overuse is, "How often, and for how long, should I apply ice?" My answer often surprises people. I tell them, "I typically wouldn't ice an area of chronic pain!" Unfortunately, regular icing seems to have become standard practice as part of an ongoing "self-care" regimen for chronic pain, especially if it stems from an acute injury. While there may be some short term relief from nagging symptoms. This approach can have long term repercussions.

    While we are all familiar with the RICE approach to treating an acute injury – **R**est, **I**ce, **C**ompression, and **E**levation - I think this protocol has been mistakenly generalized to the treatment of chronic issues. There is a time and place for therapeutically icing an injury, however in Traditional Chinese Medicine (TCM) it is used sparingly and as a short term intervention. Even in Western Medicine, the protocol for icing an acute injury is for the first 48-72 hours. From a TCM perspective, *overuse* of ice, even for an acute injury, can exacerbate symptoms, and even *create* a chronic condition.

    Swelling is often considered to be "bad" and that it should be eliminated. I wonder if this idea is a response to a cultural propensity to focus on symptoms, rather than the cause of symptoms. But swelling serves a purpose! The swelling mechanism is a very important aspect of the healing process. Swelling results from nutrient and enzyme rich fluids that bathe an injured area, assisting in the healing process and providing natural "splinting" for protection. The body is so wise! If these fluids are blocked, then the healing process is impeded and the injury is more likely to become a chronic problem.

This is not to say ice should never be used. Ice can be invaluable when used in a timely and targeted manner. Certainly it can help control pain immediately following a physical trauma, or help reduce severe swelling that is cutting off circulation. The problem arises when it is used too much or for too long.

From a western medical approach, ice is thought to keep swelling and inflammation down, while heat is thought to increase inflammation. TCM teaches that ice decreases blood circulation as it reduces inflammation, while heat increases blood circulation. This is an important distinction. While the application of heat may not always be appropriate, especially if the area of concern is red or hot to the touch, it does not necessarily mean the application of ice is appropriate as an ongoing or daily treatment approach.

If the painful area is cold or stiff, then careful application of mild heat, for short periods of 15 minutes or less, may be useful to help increase the circulation of Qi and blood in the local area. This brings oxygen and needed nutrients to the injured site and flushes out acids that may have accumulated in the tissue. In this way warmth may actually assist in the reduction of swelling, as well as help prevent the development of scar tissue.

Chinese Medicine tends to look to nature to learn about the internal workings of your body. In nature, ice slows things down; it hardens. TCM maintains that your body responds to ice much the same way. Ice slows the movement of fluids and Qi (energy), decreases blood circulation, and hardens tissue. In nature, movement is essential for life. Likewise the movement of Qi and blood through the injured area of the body is also vital.

When this flow is diminished or blocked, it can lead to "stagnant" Qi and blood. This is important from a TCM perspective, because where there is stagnation - there is pain. Icing temporarily addresses the symptoms, while establishing the free flow of Qi and blood assists in the actual healing process.

So how does this apply to the person who may experience ongoing symptoms of chronic pain stemming from an injury? I stated that ice should typically be reserved for the first 24 – 48 hours of an acute injury. So when it comes to treating overuse symptoms, what is a working definition of "acute?"

Acute conditions tend to be severe and sudden in onset, while chronic conditions usually develop over time. However, it is possible to have an acute attack in the midst of a chronic syndrome, especially if there is an underlying "root" weakness in the body's energetic system, insufficient recovery time before resuming activities, or if poor ergonomics or other exacerbating factors are involved. This is the situation many face.

Even so, the continual application of ice can cause a stagnation of Qi and blood, thereby blocking the healing process. This can create and perpetuate a vicious cycle. It may be likened to someone taking Ibuprofen daily for headaches who begins to experience Ibuprofen induced "rebound" headaches. A cycle has been established which may be difficult to break.

The goal must be to address and remediate the root cause of the injury, not just symptoms of discomfort and swelling. As such, it is important to implement a multi-dimensional program designed to strengthen the body, as well as nourish and encourage the healthy flow of Qi and blood.

Acupuncture and Chinese herbs can be extremely important aspects of such a program. These modalities are designed to help harmonize and balance the flow of Qi and blood in the body. When Qi and blood are flowing freely, the body's natural healing process is engaged, and pain and swelling *naturally* decreases.

- **Eat to reduce inflammation and pain.** See Chapter 10 for details.

- **Use caution with braces.** Many interpreters wear braces daily, sometimes for hours at a time. While there is a time and place for the judicious use of braces, I find that they are used in ways that often create long term difficulties. The problem with excessive use of braces is that the muscles become dependent on the braces for support. This allows muscles to atrophy and grow weaker and create a challenge when these weaker muscles are called upon to sustain the work required for interpreting.

  I believe braces can be helpful for maintaining a neutral hand/wrist position during sleep, and when there is an acute situation requiring substantial stabilization of the area. However, I do not support long term use of braces while working. If you are unable to interpret safely without the use of a brace, taking some time off in order to recover might be called for.

Chapter 10
A Plateful of Pain - or Energy?

Food, Inflammation and Pain:

Food is intended to give pleasure, as well as nourish, strengthen and energize your body. The problem is that most of us developed eating patterns that, while satisfying taste buds, do not optimally nourish. Certain foods increase the inflammatory response and pain levels in the body.

Eating pseudo-food filled with numerous chemicals has become commonplace. Many Americans can go for weeks without so much as eating a fresh green vegetable. The problem with this pattern for sign language interpreters is that your body needs adequate nutrition in order to heal the myriad "micro traumas" and reduce the inflammation that can occur while interpreting.

It is important to minimize foods that increase the body's inflammatory response and pain levels. Some commonly eaten foods and food additives have been shown in research studies to provoke an inflammatory response, cause cellular death and increase pain levels in the body.[9]

Preventing and/or managing pain is an important topic for sign language interpreters. If there is inadequate rest and recovery time, the cumulative effects of the repetitive movements demanded by the interpreting task may put substantial strain on the muscles and tendons of the upper extremity. This can result in microscopic tears.

Additionally, tendons and their coverings, called sheaths, begin to rub together because of inadequate lubrication resulting from overuse. The tendons then become inflamed and irritated, resulting in pain, especially with movement. Along with managing the cumulative effects of repetitive motions on the body, some interpreters may also cope with other chronic inflammatory conditions such as arthritis.

As part of a comprehensive approach to pain, it can be helpful to avoid foods known to increase pain and inflammation in the body, while consuming foods that naturally inhibit inflammatory response and reduce pain. Some of the categories to consider include:

- ♣ **Excitotoxins:** Monosodium glutamate (MSG), aspartame, yeast extract, textured protein and soy protein isolate (a common ingredient in many soy-based meat substitute products) and refined sugars are among the culprits that may be implicated in the increase of pain levels in the body. These substances are considered to be "excitotoxins."

Excitotoxins are toxins known to hyper-stimulate and excite neurons, the primary cells of the nervous system. This can lead to injury, or even death, of the neurons. Additionally, these foods can cause the body to release several neuropeptides, or amino acids, two of which are "Substance P" and glutamate. Substance P is an important link in the transmission of pain signals in the body. It can also increase the body's inflammatory response that is intricately associated with pain. Glutamate functions directly as an excitotoxin.

Eating excitotoxic foods not only can increase and sharpen a person's experience of pain, but has also been shown to negatively impact a number of neurological and other disorders including fibromyalgia, migraine headaches, various skin diseases, seizures, as well as some autoimmune disorders.

- ♣ **Food and the Inflammatory response:**
  - o **Don't:** In addition to excitotoxic food eliciting an inflammatory response, arachidonic acid, commonly found in meat, eggs, and shellfish can also contribute to inflammation and pain if eaten in excessive amounts.

  - o **Do:** *Take Fish Oil* and eat other anti-inflammatory foods (unless you are allergic to fish, have a food sensitivity to fish or are on a blood thinner). Fish oil is one of the things I prescribe most to patients dealing with issues of chronic pain or inflammation. Adding flaxseed, pumpkin seeds and walnuts can help reduce arachidonic acid, and therefore inflammation.

    Some foods and spices may block enzymes known to increase pain and inflammation. These are known as anti-inflammatory foods. They include ginger, cayenne pepper, turmeric, green tea, red wine, pineapples, avocados, garlic, onions and fish oil. I think fish oil is best for those without fish allergies since the body does not have to "convert" it for use like it must do with plant based oils. If you opt to use fish oil, make sure it is heavy metal free (mercury, lead, cadmium, etc.).

    Additionally, many of the plant-based essential fatty acids are substantial sources of omega 6 and 9. Most Americans already consume too much of these.

- **Nightshades and Arthritis:** If there is an underlying arthritic condition there are several additional foods that are thought to be detrimental. They are generally known as nightshades. The most commonly consumed nightshades include white potatoes, tomatoes, eggplant, peppers (any kind) and paprika. I have seen miraculous results when people afflicted with arthritis completely eliminate these foods from their diet.

    In contrast, in Oriental Medicine, cherries are considered to be the best food therapy for arthritis. Turmeric is also extremely beneficial. These interventions can be helpful to a sign language interpreter who is experiencing arthritis, while at the same time trying to prevent or manage interpreting related symptoms.

    Avoiding foods and food additives known to increase pain and inflammation in the body, while concurrently adding foods and herbs that reduce inflammation can be an important part of a comprehensive program of preventing and managing pain. Eating foods that are natural and unprocessed is one of the easiest ways to reduce the amount of excitotoxins you consume.

- **pH Balance:** Your body should be slightly more alkaline than acidic. Ideally, it should remain within a range of 6.8 and 7.5. However many if not most of Americans fall well below that level. The ramifications of being in a chronic acidic state are significant. It impacts every system in the body. If the pH alkaline levels are too low, a condition called acidosis results. Your body's pH affects your electrolyte levels which in turn affects the assimilation of needed nutrients. Eventually this can cause weakening of the body, can provide a medium in which unhealthy cells proliferate, and will make it difficult for the body to heal.

    o The chief reason your body can become acidic is because of the intake of acid-forming foods and drinks. Some common culprits include coffee, tea, milk, soda, meat, refined sugar and fruit juices. Some common foods that help alkalinize the body include celery, raw spinach, broccoli, lemons (although they are acidic, they leave an alkaline "residue"), maple syrup, green vegetables, apples.

You can easily test your urinary pH balance using test strips purchased in your local health food store, pharmacy or off the internet.

Food and Emotions: How you eat can also impact your stress levels and emotions, thus dramatically affecting your experience of pain. There are several things I advise my patients to eat, or avoid if they are dealing with high levels of stress in their lives. What you eat affects your brain chemistry, which of course directly affects how you feel. Some considerations follow:

- **Dark Chocolate:** My patients are sometimes surprised when I tell them that a *little* dark chocolate might be good for them to add to their diet, especially if they are dealing with depression. It stimulates a variety of "feel good" chemicals and hormones that help elevate mood. It actually helps to change brain chemistry. Benefits can be seen within a few minutes to a few days, depending on the severity of the depression.

  Most people think of chocolate as the epitome of junk food. Actually, *dark* chocolate can provide some significant, proven health benefits. Dark chocolate (I usually recommend at least 65% organic dark chocolate) is chock full of flavonoids, which are natural antioxidants.

  Antioxidants help slow down the aging process, as well as reduce damaging free radicals that can lead to various diseases, including heart disease, and slow down the body's ability to heal itself. Additionally, flavonoids help lower "bad" cholesterol, and along with cocoa phenols, can assist in reducing blood pressure.

  So how much is beneficial to eat? And is milk chocolate just as good? Studies indicate only need a small amount of dark chocolate a day can help elevate mood. My experience with patients is that a little dark chocolate can work remarkably fast.

  It is important to eat only a little. More is not better. Even dark chocolate is high in calories and fat. Too much can lead to weight gain and other complications. Chocolate also has some mild stimulants that are not helpful in large amounts.

  Milk chocolate does not have the same health benefits as dark chocolate and is often higher in fat and sugar content.

- **Complex Carbohydrates:** Along with protein, complex carbs serve an important function in the production of serotonin in the brain. Serotonin is pivotal to help elevate mood. Complex carbs include *whole* grains, beans, lentils, and starchy vegetables (although white potatoes are not the best source). I have seen people start to feel significantly better within a week of drastically increasing their intake of complex carbs. As a side note, complex carbohydrates are *not* bad for you, nor do they cause weight gain. Most weight gain from carbs is due to the consumption of refined, processed carbohydrates rather than the whole, unprocessed food.

- **Protein:** Protein is essential for the production of serotonin and other chemicals in the brain necessary for healthy emotions. A good rule of thumb for calculating serving size is that your protein serving should be about the size of your open palm.

    It is important to be especially mindful of how much protein you ingest if you suffer from depression accompanied by anger and irritation. This may indicate that you are ingesting too much protein, leading to an over abundance of dopamine and norepinephrine which can lead to these types of emotions. In this situation it can be helpful to increase the consumption of complex carbohydrates and reduce the amount of protein ingested.

- **Eliminate Excitotoxins:** As mentioned above, excitotoxins hyper-stimulate and excite neurons. As well as impacting your experience of pain, it is thought by many to affect the emotions as well. I have seen tremendous improvements in the emotional health of patients who stopped or significantly reduced their intake of excitotoxins. The most common ones that I see people using are artificial sweeteners and msg.

- **Avoid smoking:** Though it is not a food, smoking is something that you take into your body which can impact your risk of IRI. When you smoke, you absorb carbon monoxide and nicotine into your body. These substances reduce the supply of oxygen to your body and brain.

    Although smoking can negatively impact your body in a variety of ways, it can also affect your risk of IRI for three reasons:

    o First, brain function is diminished when there is insufficient oxygen. This affects concentration and processing abilities. This can add tremendous stress to an interpreter.
    o Second, because muscle tissue needs oxygen in order to function in a healthy manner, smoking will increase the risk of injury, along with compromising the body's ability to heal.

- o Third, smoking is a vaso-constrictor and so reduces the circulation and availability of oxygen to your cells.

- **Caffeine:** Caffeine can potentially increase pain levels in the body. Because it is a nervous system stimulant it tends to cause increased tension in the muscles. Increased muscle tension equals increased pain.

- **Supplements:** In general, I believe supplements are a good idea if used properly. I have also seen much misuse of supplements.

  While, I think your body was intended to garner the nutrients it needs from the foods you eat, I also acknowledge that the world is not as it once was. Soil is depleted. The world is contaminated with pollutants that permeate the air, water, food and environment. Stress levels, for many, run chronically high. Since all of these things increase your need for vitamins and minerals, I think a daily supplement is helpful.

  I will not describe specific amounts here, since individual needs vary, however what I typically recommend for most adults is:

  - o A *very good* daily whole food vitamin and mineral supplement. I prefer a supplement made from whole, concentrated food.

  - o Fish oil (heavy metal free) *unless allergic, sensitive or on blood thinners (usually 1000-3000 grams)

  - o R-lipoic acid and L-carnitine. This combination is wonderful because it assists the mitochondria (the energy making cells) in creating energy for the body's use.

  - o Tart cherry juice extract for people with arthritis or other inflammatory disorders (caution for diabetics).

  - o Turmeric as an anti-inflammatory. Incidentally, there is research to indicate that turmeric may play a significant role in prevention of Alzheimer's. (Caution for ulcers or acid reflux)

  - o Chlorophyll water to help keep the PH balance of the body slightly on the alkaline side. Just a few drops will suffice. Chlorophyll can be purchased at your local health food store.

One caution with using chlorophyll drops is that it can cause loose stools if you use too much. Just drop the amount back until your stools are formed and easily passed.

Nutrition and Oriental Medicine: Nutritional intervention to assist in healing is an important aspect of Oriental medicine.[11]   Several foods are believed to cause Qi, or energy, to become stuck or blocked in the body. This becomes significant when it is understood that where Qi does not flow, there is pain, and where there is pain, Qi is not flowing.

Foods that can cause a stagnation of Qi are:

- **Greasy foods**
- **Excessive dairy, especially cheese**
- **Cold food and drinks**
- **Refined foods and sugar**

So next time you sit down to a meal, consider making it a pain-free one... and Bon appetite!

Chapter 11

Self Care Using Acupressure and Self-Massage

Oriental medicine can be a powerful modality for self care. Learning these techniques is an empowering way to take control of your own health. However, **self-treatment is *not* intended to replace appropriate and necessary medical treatment. It can, however, effectively supplement any medical intervention.** It is a powerful preventive strategy, as well as helping you manage symptoms resulting from overuse.

The effectiveness of the treatments and the number that may be required depends on how long you have had the injury, how severe it is, and your current health status. If you have a longstanding, chronic condition, repeated treatments over a long period of time may be required. If your symptoms are mild and recent, results may be fast and more dramatic. If your condition is permanent, acupressure and self-massage may be helpful to mediate pain and stress.

Acupressure and self-massage have many significant functions including:

- **Reduces stress**

- **Releases physical muscle tension**

- **Increases blood and Qi circulation**

- **Dissipates energy blocks**

- **Stimulates production of white blood cells, thus enhancing immune function**

- **Releases natural painkillers**

- **Improves mental function**

- **Stabilizes and relaxes joints**

- **Strengthens tendons**

- ♣ **Helps the body heal faster**

- ♣ **Enhances performance**

- ♣ **Prevents future injuries**

General acupressure and self-massage strategies: Following are some helpful suggestions on how to use acupressure and self-massage:

- ♣ Massage only to the intensity of 3 out of 10. Many people think "more is better." In reality massage or acupressure that is too aggressive can exacerbate things at worst, and be ineffective at best. It is possible that the muscle tissue may rebound and spasm with an overly aggressive approach or cut off the flow of Qi. Massaging at an intensity level of 3 out of 10 is strong enough to be effective and yet not too forceful to be harmful.

- ♣ Massage each point for approximately 30 seconds on each side two to three times a day. Too much massage can lead to local bruising and excessive tenderness.

- ♣ Continue to breathe normally. Breathing allows and encourages the free flow of Qi. Ceasing to breathe can result in an increase in physical tension and stagnant Qi.

Tui Na Self Massage: Tui Na is a system of body work that has been performed as an integral part of Chinese medicine for thousands of years. Tui means to "push" and Na means "life and squeeze." Learning the basics of this time honored system can be helpful for interpreters because it empowers you with a wonderful tool for self-care.[12] Tui Na bodywork promotes muscle and joint health and mobility.

- ♣ **Tui Na includes eight primary massage techniques:**
    - o **Tui:** Pushing
    - o **Na:** Pulling or dragging
    - o **An:** Pressing
    - o **Tao:** Pinching

- o **Nie:** Kneading
- o **Nipping:** Pressing with nail
- o **Moa:** Rubbing
- o **Pai:** Tapping

There are myriad ways in which Tui Na can be used to help in the prevention and management of IRI. Some uses I have found particularly helpful for sign language interpreters include:

♣ **Every morning:**
- o **Pai** (Tap) the thymus. The thymus is located just behind your breast bone, just above your breasts. If you tap firmly about 20 times on the breastbone it can help to stimulate the thymus gland. The intensity should be firm, but not painful.

    The thymus gland is integral to the functioning of other hormonal glands in the endocrine system. I have found that thumping the thymus each morning helps to "wake up" the thymus gland, increases energy and helps to support the endocrine system.

    This technique would be contra-indicated for anyone with heart problems.

- **Pai** (Tap) very gently with fists or cupped hands the outside of your body, from top to bottom, then the inside of your arms and legs from bottom to top.

    The abdomen and head should be excluded in this technique and is contra-indicated if on blood thinners, if you bruise easily and should be avoided on any region of the body that is injured.

- ♣ **After meals:**
    - **Moa** (Rub) your stomach in clockwise circles to stimulate digestion. This is important since the muscles and sinews need nutritional support for the demands the interpreting task places on the body.

- **At night:**
  - **Hold forehead with one palm and base of skull with other while lying down.** While this is not really a Tui Na technique, I have found it very helpful in reducing stress. When you experience stress a significant amount of blood in your brain floods to the back of your head when the limbic system, or the "emotional" brain is located. Placing your hands on the back of your head and on your forehead at the same time keeps some of the blood in the fore-brain, the part that is more focused on logic and reasoning. Basically it helps to balance the reasoning center and the emotional centers of the brain.

- **Soak feet in hot water for 15 minutes prior to bed.** The temperature should be comfortably warm but not scalding. This helps to bring the energy down and out of the head. It is extremely helpful for insomnia, especially if you have trouble sleeping because you can't "turn your brain off."

♣ **General Daily Regimen:**
- **Na** (pull/drag) fingers from crown, down the side of your head to the neck.

- **Na** (pull/drag) fingers, starting on the forehead between the eyes, moving outward to the temples.

- **Na** (pull/drag) facial muscles and sinuses in a downward movement with fingers.

- **Cup closed hands over eyes.** Do not apply any pressure to the eyes with the hands.

- **Nie** (knead) your ears.

- **Nie** (knead) the nape of the neck using heel of hand. This is done by cupping the entire back of the neck with your palm, then using the heel of the hand to massage. To do both sides, you will need to change hands.

- **Na** (pull/drag) fingers from back of shoulders to front.

- **Pai** (tapping) shoulders lightly using tips of fingers or brush bristles. This helps to break up stuck Qi and allow for its free flow. Often people experience significant relief from tight shoulders using this technique.

- **Tui** (Push) and **Nie** (knead) arms working from shoulder to hands.

- **Tao** (Pinch) and **Nie** (knead) hands. Sometimes this can be done with oil or lotion.

- **Gently grasp shoulder and arm muscles and gently shake.** I have found that gently holding and shaking a muscle is the fastest way to get it to relax. Within just a few seconds there is often a significant release.

- **Nie** (knead) back muscles and buttocks. Sometimes I recommend people use tennis balls for this. Unless it is painful you may be able to lie down on the balls or sometimes you can tie two tennis balls in a pair of knee highs with a knot between the balls, place them on a wall and lean into them with your back, while moving your body up and down.

- **An** (Press) and **Nie** (knead) legs working from your hips to your feet.

- **Nie** (knead) foot. Some parts of the foot are easier to massage if you link your fingers between your toes and use the palm of your hand.

Mirror points: Mirror points are points on the *opposite* extremities from the side of the body experiencing symptoms. For example, if someone comes to me with wrist pain, I may treat their wrist by inserting an acupuncture needle in the ankle on the opposite side. This type of treatment is extremely effective and can be done with massage as well. In order to treat mirror points:

- ♣ **Determine area of pain**

- **Identify which extremity should be massaged in order to treat the area of pain.** The corresponding areas are (See Figure 3):
    - Hip/ankle
    - Shoulder/ankle
    - Shoulder/hip
    - Knee/elbow
    - Knee/knee
    - Wrist/ankle

Figure 3

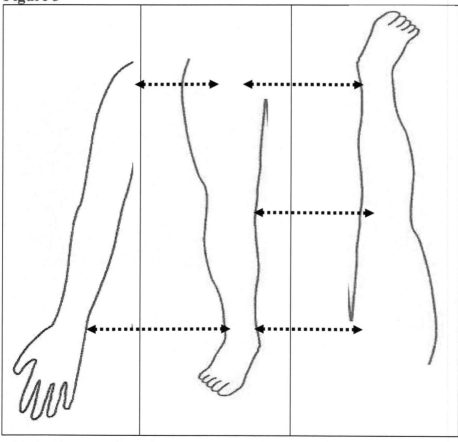

- **Always treat the opposite side of the body**

- **The extremity you will be massaging represents the one being treated.** For example, if the pain is on the thumb side of the right wrist, then massage the big toe side of the left ankle. In other words imagine where the point to treat your wrist would be on your ankle if you ankle were actually your wrist. Basically you "overlay" a template of the extremity that is in pain onto the extremity you are massaging.

- **Search for sore areas on the extremity you are massaging.** While you will be able to identify the general area to target for massage by eyeballing it, the tender points are the specific areas to be massaged.

- **Move the extremity around that is experiencing the symptoms while simultaneously massaging the limb on the opposite side to get the desired effect.**

- **Continue stimulating the point and moving the limb for one-two minutes and then move to another point.**

Hand Micro System: There are a variety of micro systems in acupuncture; however I want to focus on the micro system of the hand. For interpreters it can be a wonderful tool for self care. The areas of the hand that are germane for interpreters are the middle fingers and ring fingers. The middle finger represents the head, neck, shoulders and scapular regions. The ring finger represents the hand, wrist, elbow and shoulder areas. The palmer aspect is the front of the body and the back of the hand is the back of the body. It is very important to note that, unlike mirror points, hand micro system points always treat the same side. This means that if the right wrist is hurting you treat points on the right ring finger. The same principles on how to find the specific sore points with mirror points should be followed here. The only difference is that the same side is treated. Some helpful hints are:

- The first joint (closest to the tip of the finger) on the middle finger represents the junction between the head and neck. Often this is a great place to treat when there is neck pain.

- The area between the first and second joint of the middle finger is the neck.

- The scapular region is represented by the area between the second and last joint of the middle finger.

- The first joint (closest to the tip) of the ring finger represents the wrist.
    - The second joint of the ring finger corresponds to the elbow.
    - The last joint of the ring finger is the shoulder joint, so obviously the webbing area between the last joint of the ring finger and the middle finger is the area of the trapezius, or shoulder muscles.

Helpful Massage Points: (Note: the abbreviations assigned to the points e.g. GB20, SJ3, etc.) refer to the identity of the energy channel and the specific point on that channel. So GB20 would refer to the twentieth point along the Gall Bladder energy channel. (For the purposes of this book that level of depth will not be explored and is not necessary to locating and utilizing the points for the purpose of self care.)

See Figure 4 below for graphic depiction of point location. Point descriptions and explanations are also listed below. Generally you will find the points will be slightly tender. There may even be a small depression where the point is found.

Measurements are designated by Cuns (an ancient measurement). One Cun is equivalent to the measurement from the tip of your thumb to the first knuckle. Cuns are used because one person's body proportions will be different from another person's.

Self treatment using acupressure points:

NECK:

- **GB20:** On the nape, in the two depressions at the base of the skull below the occipital area.

- **GB39:** On the lateral (outside) aspect of the calf, 3 cun above the tip of the outside ankle bone, in front of the border of the fibula bone.

- ♣ **SI3:** When making a loose fist the point is found at the end of the crease on the side of your hand near the little finger.

- ♣ **UB60:** On the foot, directly behind the outside ankle bone, in the depression between the ankle bone and the tendon. (note: This point is contra-indicated for pregnant women)

- ♣ **SJ5:** On the back of the forearm (not palm side), two cun above the wrist between the bones on the arm.

SHOULDER:

- ♣ **SJ5:** On the back of the forearm (not palm side), two cun above the wrist between the bones on the arm.

- ♣ **LI4:** On the back of the hand, on a sore spot in the webbing between the 1st pointer finger and the thumb. (note: This point is contra-indicated for pregnant women)

- ♣ **ST12:** In the midpoint of the hollow above the clavicle, 4 cun from the midline of the body. (note: This point is contra-indicated for pregnant women)

- ♣ **ST38:** On the front aspect of the lower leg, 8 cun below the knee, one finger-breadth (middle finger) to the outside of the shinbone.

- ♣ **GB21:** On the trapezius part of the shoulder, directly above the nipple. This is usually the highest point of the trapezius muscle. (note: This point is contra-indicated for pregnant women)

- ♣ **LI15 and SJ14:** These points are found on the shoulder joint. They are two depressions right on the shoulder joint.

ELBOW:

- ♣ **SJ5:** On the back of the forearm (not palm side), two cun above the wrist between the bones on the arm.
- ♣ **LI4:** On the back of the hand, on a sore spot in the webbing between the 1st pointer finger and the thumb. (note: This point is contra-indicated for pregnant women.)

- ♣ **SI8:** This point is found in the depression on the "funny bone" of the elbow.

- ♣ **LI11:** With the elbow bent, the point is at the end of the crease on the outside aspect of the arm.

- ♣ **LI12:** With the elbow bent the point is on the outside aspect of the arm, 1 cun above LI11, on the border of the arm bone.

- ♣ **LU5:** On the crease of the elbow, in the depression just on the outside aspect of the large tendon.

WRIST:

- ♣ **ST36:** On the front aspect of the lower leg, 3 cun below the bottom of the knee, one fingerbreadth to the outside of the shinbone.

- ♣ **SP5:** In the depression below and just to the front of the inside ankle bone.

- ♣ **GB40:** In the depression below and just to the front of the outside ankle bone.

- ♣ **PC7:** Directly in the middle of the wrist crease, on the palm side of the wrist.

- ♣ **LI5:** On the thumb side of the wrist in the large depression at the base of the thumb.

- ♣ **SJ4:** On the crease on the back aspect of the wrist, in the depression on the little finger side of the tendon. This point is just off center from the midpoint of the back of the wrist.

- ♣ **SI4 and SI5:** These two points can be found on the little finger side of the wrist. The points are in depressions just below and just above the wrist crease on the side of the wrist.

FINGERS:

♣ **SJ3:** On the back of the hand, in the depression between the ring finger and little finger and just above the knuckles.

♣ **LI3:** When a loose fist is made, this point is in the fleshy depression on the thumb side of the pointer finger.

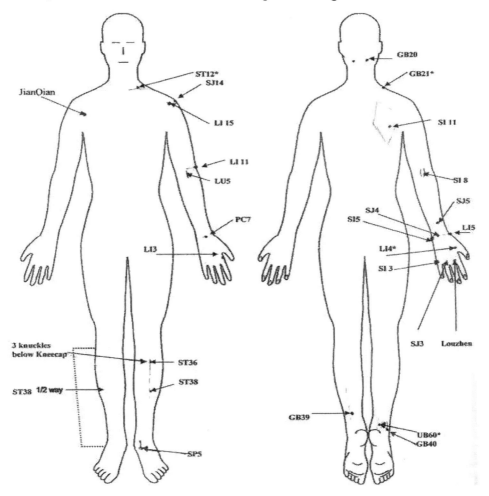

Figure 4

Chapter 12
Work Stations

Footrests:

When you have to sit at a station for a long period of time, such as in a VRS call center, there should be a footstool at each workstation. The footrest should allow for independent height and angle adjustments. This will allow each interpreter to find the position of the legs and feet best for them. Thighs should ideally be parallel to the floor or only slightly angled down when seated properly.

It is important to take care not to use the footrest to compensate for a chair that is too high. Sometimes people try to use footrests to substitute for a lower chair and/or workstation. When an interpreter inappropriately uses a footrest to compensate for inappropriate chairs or workstation heights, awkward leg postures may result. Make sure the foot doesn't rest on sharp or hard edges. Big footrests give more choice of leg posture. Footrests should be stable enough to stay in place but easy to move with the feet and legs to reposition if needed.

Chairs:

There are several features that are important to consider with chairs. Generally, if a chair is intended to meet the needs of a number of different body sizes and shapes it is helpful to have a wide variety of options and features. Some helpful features include:

- ♣ **Seat height adjustability-** Pneumatic adjustability is easier to use than mechanical. This is important in order to compensate for interpreters of different heights and for easy and fast adjustments.

- ♣ **Seat depth adjustability** – This changes the front-to-back depth of the seat either by backrest in-out adjustability or a sliding seat pan. A shorter seat pan allows smaller people to use the chair's backrest, while a deeper one feels more stable to taller individuals.

- ♣ **Backrest angle adjustability-**The ability to change the angle of the backrest.

- **Chair tilt:** The angle of the entire seat relative to the floor. A reclined chair transfers some upper-body weight to the backrest of the chair.

- **Seat pan angle adjustability:** Changing the forward-back angle of the seat. This feature provides forward tilt, in which the thighs slope downward.

- **Armrests:** I would not recommend armrests at all. Interpreters often use the arms to rest the elbow which can instigate elbow pain. Additionally chairs with arms seem to contribute to higher risk interpreting ergonomics. I have also found that when interpreters rest their arms on the chair arm it pushes their entire upper arm and shoulder upward, increasing tension and static loading in the shoulder region.

- **Lumbar support:** Helps to minimize the flattening of the lumbar spine when seated. If the lumbar support is not adjustable though, different sized people will have the "bump" hit them at different places in the back and may cause discomfort.

- **Backrest height adjustability:** This refers to a change in height of the lumbar support area of the chair backrest. This feature accommodates preferences by different interpreters regarding where and how the lumbar support curve contacts the back.

- **Lumbar depth adjustability:** This allows for adjustment of the size and sometimes the firmness of the lumbar support curve. Like backrest height adjustability, it accommodates different preferences and body shapes.

Desks:

- If desks are used they should be height adjustable using an automatic rather than manual mechanism.

Cameras:

- Monitors and the cameras should ideally be separate.

Monitors:

- ♣ Optimal distance is 20-30 inches.

- ♣ Monitor should be directly in front of you (height) and aligned so that the top row of characters on the screen is at or slightly below eye level.

Chapter 13
Making Your Body Your Ally

If you are an interpreter experiencing symptoms of overuse, you may find yourself at times feeling as though you are in an adversarial relationship with your own body. You may even find yourself using language such as "my bad arm" or "my no-good hand." While it can be frustrating when life is so profoundly affected by pain from overuse, it is important to remember that your body is not your enemy. In truth, your body constantly works very hard on your behalf. You are actually "hard-wired" to heal; it is your default programming.

You can, however, significantly impact your ability to heal by how you view and treat your body. If you see your body as an enemy, treat it with neglect, deny it adequate amounts of sleep and rest, feed it food filled with toxins rather than needed nutrients, and get little to no exercise, then you burden your body and healing is compromised. If you view your body as your ally, treat it with compassionate regard, balance your sleep and rest with appropriate levels of activity, and consume nutritious foods and sufficient water, then you support your body's natural propensity to heal.

In my practice of oriental medicine, I treat many people for overuse injuries. While acupuncture and oriental medicine is quite helpful for a variety of overuse symptoms, the prognosis for each patient also depends on their willingness to befriend their body and attend to its needs. I call this making your body your ally. I have found that there are some crucial factors that are essential in order to make your body your ally. These are:

1. Recognize that your body constantly works on your behalf to heal. It is not against you and it is not your enemy. When you view parts of your body as "bad" or "broken" or "no good," then you automatically create an adversarial relationship with your body. This is not conducive to healing.

    In recent years there has been some ground-breaking research that demonstrates our thoughts impact our capacity to heal. If you send angry, hateful thoughts or sentiments to parts of yourself that are in pain, you only add to that pain. It is not much different than getting angry at a child in pain. Anger will not assuage the child's pain, but most likely will increase his or her anguish. When you experience pain, your body is doing what it is supposed to do; it is letting you know that something is wrong and asking you for help.

2. Take a positive approach with your body and healing. Instead of saying, "my bad arm," try saying "the arm in the process of healing." Ask yourself what you can do to show compassion to the part of your body that is in pain.

3. Honor and support your body by providing it the basic essentials that are required for health. This includes nutritious food, adequate water, moderate exercise and restful sleep.

4. Foster fulfilling and intimate relationships in your life. People who have meaningful relationships live longer, healthier lives.

5. Give your body time to heal if you are experiencing an overuse injury. Making sure you give your body sufficient recovery time to heal from an overuse injury will often prevent long term consequences. It is important to listen and respond to your body's needs. In this way you can become an ally to your body and support it as it heals.

6. Listen to your body as it "talks" to you. If you listen and respond, then you will develop a strong alliance and sense of trust with your body. And your body will trust you because you respond to its needs!

7. **Do not** sacrifice your body on the altar of interpreting. Build time into your schedule to allow your body time to heal if that is what it needs. Taking care of your body is a primary professional responsibility.

8. Warming up before interpreting, and cooling down afterward is a gift to your body. It is a gentle and caring way to help your body adjust to the physical demands of interpreting.

Your body works ceaselessly for your good. Listening to your body and becoming aware of its needs is imperative for good health - however it is only a first step. Once you have the awareness, then action needs to be taken in order to correct any imbalance. Signals of discomfort communicated by the body are not much different than a good friend and neighbor pounding on your door at 2AM to let you know your house is on fire. If you get mad at the neighbor and turn over and go back to sleep, your house may burn down – with you in it! Your friend is doing you a service by pounding on your door. So too is your body.

INTERPRETER BILL OF RIGHTS

I have the right to take care of myself as my first professional responsibility.

I have the right to take reasonable breaks to allow my body to rest from interpreting.

I have the right to acknowledge and communicate my limitations and needs to myself and other appropriate individuals.

I have the right to refuse an assignment that I feel is unsafe for me or that is beyond my current ability to do with quality.

I have the right to produce work that is consistent and of quality without the expectation that I must be perfect.

I have the right to ask for what I need in order to do my work safely and with quality.

I have the right to continue to grow and develop as a professional in my field.

I have the right to make decisions about what is right for me.

I have the right to be treated with respect and as a professional. As such, I have the right to establish healthy boundaries regarding how I will be treated by consumers and employers.

I have the right to be a person *and* an interpreter at the same time.

I have the right to find satisfaction in my work.

Sources:

1. Rochester Institute of Technology (2008, April 19). Sign Language Interpreters at High Ergonomic Risk.

2. Bureau of Labor Statistics, U.S. Department of Labor, Survey of Occupational Injuries and Illnesses in cooperation with participating State agencies, Reissue date: 2009

3. Stuckless, Avery and T. Alan Hurwitz, eds. 1989. Educational interpreting for deaf students: report of the task force on educational interpreting. New York: National Technical Institute for the Deaf, Rochester Institute of Technology.

4. DeCaro, James J., Michael Feuerstein, and T. Alan Hurwitz. "Cumulative trauma disorders among educational interpreters." American Annals of the Deaf 137 (1992): 288-292

5. Feuerstein, Michael, and Terence E. Fitzgerald. "Bio-mechanical factors affecting upper extremity cumulative trauma disorders in sign language interpreters." Journal of Occupational Medicine 34 (1992): 257-264

6. Lynn S. Bickley. Bates Guide to Physical Examination and History Taking, Eight Edition, Lippincott Williams and Wilkins, 2002

7. Cumulative Trauma Disorder, Rochester Institute of Technology, 2005

8. Maoshing Ni, The Yellow Emperor's Classic of Medicine: A New Translation of the Neijing Suwen with Commentary, Shambahala Publications, 1995

9. Hyman, Mark M.D. The UltraMind Solution, Scribner Publishing (A division of Simon & Schuster, Inc), 2009

10. L. Zhang, M. Fiala, J. Cashman, et al., Curcuminoids enhance amyloid-ß uptake by macrophages of Alzheimer's disease patients. J Alzheimers Dis, 2006, vol. 10, pp. 1—7

11. Flaws, Bob. The Tao of Healthy Eating, Blue Poppy Press, 7th printing 2005

12. Xu Xiangcau. Chinese Tuina Massage: The Essential Guide to Treating Injuries, Improving Health, and Balancing Qi. YMMA Publication Center, Boston, MA., 2002

Other Resources:

Akabas, S.H., L.B. Gates, and D.E. Galvin. Disability management: A complete guide to reduce costs, increase productivity, meet employee needs, and ensure legal compliance. New York, NY: American Management Association, 1992

Caponigro, Andy. The Miracle of the Breath: Mastering Fear, Healing Illness, and Experiencing the Divine. New World Library, 2005

Cohn, Lester, Rhonda M. Lowry, and Sandra Hart. "Overuse syndromes of the upper extremity in interpreters for the deaf." Orthopedics (1989): 207-209

Crouch, Tammy, and Michael Madden. Carpal Tunnel Syndrome and Overuse Injuries. Berkley: North Atlantic Books, 1992
Cumulative Trauma Disorder – CTD, Published by The Rochester Institute of Technology, 1996

Deadman, Peter, and Baker, Kevin, A Manual of Acupuncture, Journal of Chinese Medicine Publications, 2007

Emmons, Henry and Krantz, Rachel. The Chemistry of Joy, Fireside Publishing, 2006

Feuerstein, Michael, and P.F. Hickey. "Ergonomic approaches in the clinical assessment of occupational musculoskeletal disorders." In Handbook of pain assessment, edited by D.C. Turk and R. Melzack, 71-99. New York: Guilford Press, 1992

Feldenkrais, Moshe. Awareness Through Movement: Easy-to-Do Health Exercises to Improve Your Posture Vision Imagination and Personal Awareness, Reprint Edition Paperback (Harper San Francisco; Apr 1 1991

Feuerstein, Michael. "A multidisciplinary approach to the prevention, evaluation, and management of work disability." Journal of Occupational Rehabilitation 1 (1991): 5-11

Hans-Ulrich Hecker, Angelika Steveling, and Elmar Peuker. Microsystems Acupuncture: The Complete Guide: Ear - Scalp - Mouth – Hand, Thieme International Publishing, 2005

HR World Editors, "The Ultimate Guide to Workstation Ergonomics: 10 Easy Tips", October 1, 2007

Kapchuck, Ted. The Web That Has No Weaver, Contemporary Books, 2000

Perricone, Nicholas M.D. The Perricone Promise, Warner Books, 2004

Putz-Anderson, Vern, ed. 1988. Cumulative trauma disorders: a manual for musculoskeletal diseases of the upper limbs. London: Taylor and Francis

Sanderson, Gary. "Repetitive Motion Injury." (videotape). Sign Media, Inc.

Stanford University, http://www.stanford.edu/dept/EHS/prod/general/ergo/

Stone, W.E. "Occupational repetitive strain injuries." Australian Family Physician 13 (1984): 682

National Institute of Health. "For Parents: Why Sleep is Important. http://www.nhlbi.nih.gov/health/public/sleep/starslp/parents/whysleep.hml

University Of Maryland. "Sleep Hygiene: Helpful Hints to Help You Sleep"
http://www.umm.edu/sleep/sleep_hyg.html

About The Author:

Diane Gross, DOM (NM), Dipl. OM, L.Ac. CI and CT is a Doctor of Oriental Medicine (NM), licensed acupuncturist and certified sign language interpreter. In addition to working in a highly successful and busy acupuncture clinic in Greensboro, NC, she also serves as a nationally recognized sign language interpreting ergonomic consultant, specializing in providing instruction and diagnostics for interpreters seeking to reduce or manage their risk of interpreting related pain and injury.

Diane served as Project Coordinator and senior writer in the development of training materials on the prevention and management of interpreting related injury for the National Technical Institute of Technology (NTID) in the early 1990s. Since that time she has continued to provide workshops and assessments for interpreters across the country.

While most "generalist" ergonomic experts have been only marginally successful in helping interpreters because they don't know sign language, Diane is especially adept in assisting and training interpreters, since she is skilled both in sign language and interpreting ergonomics. She also brings a unique perspective on self-care using principles based in Oriental Medicine, acupressure, self-massage and nutritional interventions.

Diane is currently the managing practitioner at Stillpoint Acupuncture, located in North Carolina, as well as the owner of TerpHealth$_{TM}$. She utilizes her extensive knowledge of ergonomics, energy medicine, nutrition and Oriental Medicine with her patients and clients with ongoing success.

Diane's TerpHealth$_{TM}$ website is **www.TerpHealth.com.** She can be contacted through the website. She also regularly posts on her Facebook page TerpHealth. Books authored by her may be ordered at **www.createspace.com**

Made in the USA
Charleston, SC
26 August 2015